Nursing: Images and Ideals

Opening Dialogue with the Humanities

Stuart F. Spicker, Ph.D., a philosopher, is Professor of Community Medicine and Health Care at the University of Connecticut School of Medicine, Farmington. He is coeditor of the book series *Philosophy and Medicine*, an associate editor of the newly founded journal *Meta-medicine*, and consulting editor for the series "Humanistic Studies in Medicine" in *Connecticut Medicine*.

Sally Gadow, R.N., Ph.D., a nurse/philosopher, is Assistant Professor in the Department of Community Health and Family Medicine, College of Medicine, University of Florida, Gainesville. During 1978-1979 she was the recipient of a Joseph P. Kennedy, Jr., Founda-tion Fellowship for the Study of Ethics and Nursing at the Kennedy Institute of Ethics, Georgetown University, Washington, D.C.

NURSING: IMAGES AND IDEALS

Opening Dialogue with the Humanities

Stuart F. Spicker, Ph.D.
Sally Gadow, R.N., Ph.D.
Editors

WITH ELEVEN CONTRIBUTORS

SPRINGER PUBLISHING COMPANY
New York

Copyright © 1980 by Stuart F. Spicker, Ph.D.

Springer Publishing Company, Inc.
200 Park Avenue South
New York, N.Y. 10003

80 81 82 83 84 / 10 9 8 7 6 5 4 3 2 1

Library of Congress Cataloging in Publication Data

Main entry under title:

Nursing, images and ideals.

   Includes bibliographical references and index.
   Selected essays from a conference initiated by
the Committee on Philosophy and Medicine, American
Philosophical Association and held at the University
of Connecticut Health Center in Farmington.
   1. Nursing—Philosophy—Congresses. 2. Nursing
ethics—Congresses. I. Spicker, Stuart F., 1937-
II. Gadow, Sally. III. American Philosophical
Association. Committee on Philosophy and Medicine.
RT84.5.N87   610.73'01   79-15057
ISBN 0-8261-2740-1
ISBN 0-8261-2741-X pbk.

Printed in the United States of America

This publication was made possible by a grant from The Massachusetts Foundation for the Humanities and Public Policy. We acknowledge with gratitude the material support of the Foundation and in particular we wish to thank Nathaniel Reed, Ph.D., the Executive Director of the Foundation, for his encouragement and assistance in enabling us to bring this volume before the public.

S.F.S.
S.G.

Contents

Contributors

NATALIE ABRAMS, Ph.D., is Assistant Professor of Philosophy, Philosophy and Medicine Program, New York University Medical School, New York City.

MILA ANN AROSKAR, R.N., Ed.D., is Associate Professor, Department of Public Health Nursing, School of Public Health, The University of Minnesota, Minneapolis.

ROBERT BAKER, Ph.D., is Assistant Professor of Philosophy, Department of Philosophy, Union College, Schenectady, New York.

BERTRAM BANDMAN, Ph.D., is Professor of Philosophy, Department of Philosophy, Long Island University, Brooklyn Center, New York City.

ELSIE BANDMAN, R.N., Ed.D., is Professor, Hunter College—Bellevue School of Nursing, New York City.

DAN W. BROCK, Ph.D., is Associate Professor of Philosophy, Department of Philosophy, Brown University, Providence, Rhode Island.

SANDRA HARDING, Ph.D., is Assistant Professor of Philosophy, Department of Philosophy, University of Delaware, Newark, Delaware.

JOHN LADD, Ph.D., is Professor of Philosophy, Department of Philosophy, Brown University, Providence, Rhode Island.

LISA NEWTON, Ph.D., is Professor of Philosophy, Department of Philosophy, Fairfield University, Fairfield, Connecticut.

SHERI SMITH, Ph.D., is Associate Professor of Philosophy, Department of Philosophy, Rhode Island College, Providence.

KATHLEEN M. SWARD, R.N., Ed.D., is Professor of Nursing and Director of the Nursing Program, Elmira College, Elmira, New York.

Preface

This collection of essays by nurses and philosophers on ethical issues in the profession and practice of nursing is the outcome of a project conceived in Boston in December, 1976, at the Seventy-Third Annual Meeting of the Eastern Division of the American Philosophical Association. During that meeting the Committee on Philosophy and Medicine convened to discuss its interests, goals, and future projects. Chairman of the Committee John Ladd, Professor of Philosophy at Brown University, informed the membership that he had received a number of letters encouraging the Committee to establish dialogue between nurses and philosophers. Professors of philosophy had written expressing their interest in pursuing issues and problems germane to the profession and practice of nursing. In a few instances philosophers were actively involved in nursing education and a few nurses were undertaking graduate work in philosophy, specifically focusing their dissertations on ethical issues in nursing and health care.

Nurses have for some time been attending regional and national meetings on bioethics. At the meeting of the Committee on Philosophy and Medicine the nurses in attendance encouraged a unique meeting with philosophers, a project involving dialogue among nurses, philosophers and the public, with special attention to what the philosophers might learn about the profession and practice of nursing, both within and outside of nursing academe. On March 4-5, 1977, a group of twenty-four humanists and nurses convened at the University of Connecticut Health Center in Farmington. This planning session and the subsequent project were supported equally by grants from four state humanities committees of the National Endowment for the Humanities: The Connecticut Humanities Council (P7710-G7716); The Massachusetts Foundation for Humanities and Public Policy (May 7-2); The New York Council for the Humanities (77-301); and The Rhode Island Committee for the Humanities (767721). These four grant awards made an annual project possible; the project was conducted in three phases: (1) a regional three-day conference in November, 1977, at which philosophers and nurses could together explore the focal issues in nursing which had bearing on ethical decision-making from the point of view of the nurse; (2) twenty-two meetings throughout Connecticut, Massachusetts, New York, and Rhode Island at which the public could become acquainted with some of the salient issues facing the nursing profession, with philosophers serving as mediators in the exchange of ideas (total attendance at these sessions exceeded 2,300 persons); (3) a final workshop-conference held at The University of Connecticut Health Center in November, 1978, attended by persons who could pursue the goals of the project beyond the region and into nursing schools and community-based nursing practice.

This volume of essays is based upon a selection of the focal papers and commentaries presented at the initial conference in November, 1977, and reflects the commitment among philosophers and nurses to deal with the ethical issues confronting the nursing profession.

Given the long tradition of the oppression of women and the fact that women constitute 97 percent of the nursing profession, the time is propitious to address those issues which have yet to be confronted openly and articulated in the public arena. The long-standing concern of philosophy is to assist in the process of emancipation and to counterargue and counteract all forms of servitude, especially where it is most subtly at work and accepted as the "natural" attitude, apparently in need of no reflection or social critique. This project, especially the essays in this collection, seeks to unveil the assumptions, values, and stereotypes which have contributed to the long subjugation of the nurse. Historical images, modern ethical dilemmas, and ideals for future development and practice are explored in the endeavor to illuminate—for both the public and the profession—the crucial transition occurring in nursing as it moves away from its position of political and intellectual subordinance.

The fundamental assumption on which we based the entire project was the belief that there exists an important range of issues which philosophers until recently have failed to explore, having focused their attention on "medical ethics,"—that is, ethical issues in medicine, issues facing physicians, not nurses. In this collection of essays nurses and philosophers refine the issues and illuminate ethical dilemmas in nursing.

This volume, then, is largely the product of the efforts of many persons who participated in the initial phase of "Nursing and the Humanities: A Public Dialogue," working under the informal rubric "The Four-State Consortium for Nursing and the Humanities." The Consortium was led by state-coordinators—nurses and philosophers—all of whom worked extremely hard to bring about a successful project. My thanks to Anne Donnelly and Lisa Newton of Connecticut; Howard Hunter and Catherine Murphy of Massachusetts; Elsie Bandman, Peter Williams, and Bertram Bandman of New York; Lois Monteiro and Sheri Smith of Rhode Island. In addition, I extend my appreciation to Teresa Christy, Carleton Dallery, Ellen Fahy, and Sally Gadow, all of whom served as consultants to the project. In particular, the Project Director and Editors wish to offer their gratitude to Gail Fitzgerald, whose indefatigable labors with and meticulous devotion to the project and volume were indispensable to their completion.

The project was a complex one, being regional in design and execution. Such complexity required the competent, cooperative efforts of the Executive Directors of four state humanities committees, which function under the Division of State Programs of the National Endowment for the Humanities. My personal appreciation is warmly extended to Marianne Barnaby Finnegan (Connecticut), Nathaniel Reed (Massachusetts), Ronald Florence and Carol Groneman (New York), and Thomas Roberts (Rhode Island).

This collection is largely the outcome of the work of Sally Gadow, who is mainly responsible for its conception and the imaginative organization of the essays. The contributors responded with grace and promptness in supplying the revisions based on consultation with Sally Gadow and her useful editorial suggestions. For any errors of commission or omission, I take full responsibility, but credit for all that is good in this volume must go to my co-editor and the authors.

Stuart F. Spicker
Project Director

Introduction

It is a fundamental premise of nursing that a patient has the right to receive affirmation and acknowledgment as a human being. Human beings are unique and so complex that each individual transcends the categories of science. Thus, the recipient of nursing care has more than a legal right to scientific and technically competent treatment—the patient has a moral right to humanistic care.

This right is addressed by the humanities within the health-care professions. The humanities are concerned not only with understanding the depth and scope of human experience, but with creating or uncovering more human meanings for experience. Thus the humanities are engaged not only in providing illuminating, heuristic images, but in formulating ideals as well. The words "ideal" and "more human meaning" mean a way of understanding an experience that enhances its value for the individual and enables that person to formulate a meaning that uniquely expresses his or her relation to the experience. The moral right to humanistic health care is, accordingly, the right to receive from health professionals assistance in determining the personal value and meaning of one's illness or disability.

A project that attempts to address humanistic issues in nursing in a systematic manner is perhaps the most fundamental way to acknowledge that right. The value of such inquiry, however, depends greatly upon the initial identification of issues. The haphazard selection of problems and topics on the basis of current movements, popular causes, or controversial court decisions will inevitably ignore some issues and overemphasize others.

If we think of the humanities and nursing as two participants in a dialogue, two possibilities for more methodic delineation of nursing issues suggest themselves. One method is to identify and organize issues from the side of the humanities, that is, according to the distinct approaches to human experience that the humanities represent: the philosophical, the historical, and the esthetic. The second possibility is to delineate issues from the side of nursing and then determine which of the several approaches of the humanities offers the clearest elucidation. While it is the second of these methods of organization to which the present volume aspires, at times it follows the first more closely.

In looking at nursing from the three humanities perspectives that can be distinguished—the historical, the esthetic, and the philosophical—one can identify different areas of concern. The historical approach focuses on the origin and evolution of present values and coming changes in nursing. Thus the use of historical studies would be especially relevant in examining and criticizing, for example, health-care systems. The esthetic approach, with its focus upon the unique, nonquantifiable dimensions of human experience, would appropriately address such issues as the subjective and expressly individual aspects of the experience of illness as portrayed, for example, in literature. Finally, the philosophical approach, often the only one employed in humanities teaching in health-care settings, addresses issues of the moral permissibility of certain practices, as well as the more difficult issues of, not right and wrong, but permissible versus ideal ways of caring for persons. Beyond these ethical issues, philosophy is also concerned with questions about the nature of humanness and the fundamental forms of human relating; thus it would address, for example, the issue of which particular form of relation constitutes the basis for the nurse-patient relation.

The second method is that of delineating issues from the side of nursing, rather than through the humanities approaches. This method seems the more useful tool in identifying the so-called humanistic issues for the following reason. There is no division in nursing (or in any human services profession) between humanistic and nonhumanistic issues. The principal elements of the nursing process are persons, and thus the human, nontechnical, value dimensions are by definition an essential aspect of the practice of nursing. There is, in other words, *no element of nursing that is without humanistic issues*. In seeking to identify those issues, then, a natural method seems to be to lift out *all* of the fundamental issues in nursing, on the assumption that all of them are in principle humanistic. The next step would be to explore the ways in which each of those issues can be most appropriately addressed and elucidated by one or more of the humanities approaches. Since the important components of the practice of nursing are the human beings involved, a natural organization of issues, based upon the various interrelations of those persons, suggests itself. The issues would thus cluster in this way, emerging around these relations:

1. The nurse and the patient (the term "patient" is used here simply from custom, rather than as a resolution in advance of the important issues reflected in the range of terms now in use, from "patient" and "client" to "consumer")
2. The nurse and other health professionals
3. Nurses and nursing
4. The nurse and the community

Some of the specific issues within each of these categories and the particular humanities approaches that might address them are outlined below.

THE NURSE AND THE PATIENT

Defining the nurse-patient relation

What are the historical and the present forms of the nurse-patient relation and what is the ideal relation to which both nurses and the public would agree and aspire? The possibilities are not unfamiliar to anyone who has provided or received nursing care: the nurse as parent surrogate, healer, physician surrogate, contracted clinician, patient advocate, health educator, or provider of some unique and yet undefined type of care falling within none of the stereotypic nurse-patient relations, or finally, a grand and unique synthesis of all of the above.

One approach to this issue is a phenomenological inquiry into the experience of illness, to elucidate the distinction between the body as an external object and the body as a lived interiority. The implications of that distinction for nursing are becoming apparent. To cite one example: studies by nurse-researcher Dr. Jean Johnson have shown that postoperative patients were affected more positively (less analgesia, shorter hospital stay, etc.) when given preoperative information about the subjective sensations that they might experience after surgery than when given a description of the objective phenomenon they would undergo, namely, the surgical procedure. The question of whether nursing should ideally address the individual as a lived subjective body, an organ-system/object-body, or a unity of the two surely has implications for the nature of the nurse-patient relation.

A second philosophical concern with the body and illness is the issue of the value of suffering, or the religion of health. Existentialists maintain that we are free to determine the meaning that any experience will have for us, no matter how anguished or unfree we feel. Nietzsche makes a still stronger claim that pain is a positive, even necessary, means of finding one's own way, of creating oneself, and the sympathy of those who rush to comfort us only devalues our experience. The question then of whether suffering is a defect of human existence or a uniquely human possibility for self-determination is an issue that nursing must address. If suffering is an experience the meaning of which must be decided by each individual (unencumbered by the health professions' negative value of illness), the task of the nurse then becomes infinitely complex—to assist each patient in an individual manner to establish the particular meaning that his or her suffering is to have.

In addition to the approaches of phenomenology and existential philosophy, the perspective of history is essential to help clarify the extent to which the traditional role of the nurse, as a steadfastly caring and minimally technical person, has been a function of the level of technology involved in health care. Without question, the role of the modern nurse requires far more knowledge and skill concerning equipment and apparatus than ever before. Does the advancement of technology in nursing signify a necessary concomitant: a decline in the customary caring that has characterized nursing? Is nursing faced with a decision between preserving its commitment to *caring*, on the one hand, and following the progress of medical science with more technically intricate *curing*, on the other hand?

Ethical Problems and the Nurse-Patient Relation

What are the moral implications of the relation that exists between nurse and patient? Are there ethical decisions that nurses should be prohibited from making, just as there are clinical or therapeutic decisions that they are not permitted to make? Or, on the contrary, do nurses have ethical responsibilities to patients that even surpass those of other professionals who are less intimately and continuously involved with the patient? A philosophical analysis of such ethical issues would have to address the fundamental nature of the relation between a person who needs care and one who assumes responsibility for rendering that care. For example, does the patient have the right to receive from the nurse information withheld by other professionals? Does the nurse, if acting as parent surrogate, have the right to act paternalistically when the patient does not make "healthy" decisions? Does the nurse, if acting in contractual partnership with the patient, have the right to withdraw care when the patient refuses to assume responsibility for his or her health? Does the nurse, if acting as healer, analogous to the physician, have the right to cultivate the placebo effect that is thought to accompany all of the actions of a healer, even to the point of deception? Or does the nurse, if acting as patient advocate, have an obligation to protect the patient from every erosion of human dignity and value, including deceptions in the name of health? Finally, if nursing is a synthesis of all of these roles, how are values reconciled when the roles conflict, as they often clearly do?

THE NURSE AND OTHER HEALTH PROFESSIONALS

The relation between nurses and their colleagues in health care has become a pressing issue because of at least two developments: the emergence of new health professions with which the traditional professions must articulate and the increasing autonomy of midlevel practitioners as physicians become willing to delegate more of their tasks and authority. The issues for nursing can be formulated in the following ways: (1) What does the increasing number of independent nurse practitioners signify for the future of nursing? Is nursing practice striving to become another version of medical practice, rather than an alternative and complementary form of care? Or are nurse pracititioners seeking to offer a true alternative to the traditional medical practitioner by providing the same general care but in a different fashion? If so, what is that difference? And why is an alternative thought to be necessary? (2) A second issue is the changing relation between nurse and physician in their roles as members of the health-care team (as distinct from their roles as independent practitioners). Nurses are becoming increasingly responsible and critical concerning the quality of care that patients receive from their physicians. Nurses challenge orders to resuscitate patients, orders not to resuscitate patients, and at times simply make decisions directly contrary to orders that they think unjustified. The nurse is, of course, professionally obligated to challenge a medically unsafe or unsound order. Is there a comparable obligation to refuse an order that is ethically indefensible in the nurse's view? Does the physician's ethical as well as medical opinion have more authority than that of the nurse (especially when the nurse is in agreement with the expressed view of the patient)? Should the nurse, in other words, be legally required to honor an order, such as the directive to continue intravenous fluids for a terminal patient—or to discontinue them—when the order is based solely on the physician's moral view of the case, as many decisions in health care are?

Here the disciplines of history, law, and moral philosophy are all needed in addressing such an involved issue as the legal, ethical, and professional divisions—past, present, and future—between nurses and other health-care providers. One approach that might prove interesting as well as bring issues quickly to the surface would be an interprofessional debate of hypothetical "right to die" legislation allowing the *nurse* to assent to a patient's request for discontinuing extraordinary, life-sustaining measures when the attending physician refuses to do so.

NURSES AND NURSING: THE
RELATION OF NURSES TO THEMSELVES
AND THEIR PROFESSION

Images of Women Healers in Art and Literature

Because 97 percent of nurses are women and because many of the issues around the nurse-patient and the nurse-physician relation are entangled with issues of women's history, as evidenced by the cliché of the nurse as mother of the patient and wife of the physician, it would seem crucial to address explicitly the relation between women and nursing. One way of clarifying that relation is by examining images of women and women healers in literature and the visual arts. Such an inquiry would constitute a historical as well as an esthetic approach because it would document the image of women that cultures have expressed through their artists, images that not only are reflected in art and literature, but also may in part be created by artists and writers.

Women in the History of Health Care

Another way of clarifying the relation between women and nursing is to examine historically the situation of women in the health sector. This would entail analyzing not only women as such, but the socio-economic and political systems that generate and perpetuate the present situation of women. If the traditional role division within the family is accepted as part of the basis for the sex hierarchy in the health sector, critical historical studies of the family are required for elucidating the so-called family structure of the health team—with its male leader, female auxiliary, and devoted dependents. On the other hand, since the study of history offers us interpretations rather than facts, it would be simplistic to conclude that the same social and economic needs that seem to have delegated the role of nurturing support to women in the family are also the reason why nursing has been traditionally a role of "motherly care." If that were the case, we would have to predict that the liberation of women will mean the liberation of nursing, but it is not clear that the caring functions of the nurse are entirely analogous to those of the mother, or that—even if they are— nurses would want to discard them for more "liberated" functions.

Holistic Nursing: Whole Nurse or Whole Patient?

It is often maintained that optimal healing depends upon the interaction of patient and professional as whole human beings. This view is then translated into concern for the patient as a unique psychobiological whole that is self-responsible and self-healing. What is lost in that translation is the professional. To what extent is the whole person of the healer—in this case the nurse—a necessary corollary for optimal healing of the whole patient? In recent years, nurses have been acutely concerned with achieving full professional stature as health-care providers. Is the commitment to professionalism antithetical to the concern for holistic, or whole person, healing of the patient? Does the patient in any way require whole-person involvement of the nurse? The distinction between personal and professional involvement has been kept carefully sharp, ostensibly for the protection of the patient. Patients now complain that their care is too impersonal. Do they mean too professional? Or are they simply responding to the movement of humanistic health care, which can be interpreted as the movement to soften the distinction between personal and professional involvement?

This issue must not be left to the humanistic psychologies, although they can surely be credited with much of the personalization of the professional. The issue requires a sound and new conceptual framework with the means for unifying and transcending the once contradictory relation between professional and personal. What seems to be needed, among other things, is a more ample and complex, and thus more human, concept of the body. Any efforts to rehumanize health care cannot be confined to a concept of the body that holds medicine to be an exact science, and the practitioner a scientist. Or, in the case of the nurse, a research assistant whose objectivity is inviolate, if at times untherapeutic. The task of addressing the problem belongs to philosophy and art. Philosophy provides a conceptual reexamination and a phenomenological rediscovery of the whole person as body, and the arts provide esthetic, nonanalytic access to human experience through images of the body that the artist portrays. A single work such as Degas' tender painting of a girl-woman sitting unclothed on a bed, bewildered, wondering, can in itself make the point that one's experience and image of one's body are so intimate and inward, and often excruciatingly fragile, that the height of dehumanization would be an objective, "professional" treatment of the body as an external object, a clinical entity.

THE NURSE AND THE COMMUNITY

Community Control: Nursing and a National Health Service

The insulation of the health industry from the needs of the community is slowly diminishing. Consumerism, plus the consciousness-raising of the public with respect to health and health care, means that all of the health professions will be held increasingly accountable for the distribution of practitioners, both in geography and in specialty, and for their professional training, particularly as it concerns the values of human dignity, quality care, and nondiscrimination. The issue for nursing is thus the extent to which the profession can and should share with the public the responsibility for adjusting the maldistribution of health workers. A related issue is whether that adjustment should extend to the very foundation of health care, namely, professional education, with the possible effect that the levels within the professional hierarchy would be equalized by educating health workers together in health-team schools, with a basic curriculum for all categories of practitioners and with control of admissions and curriculum for all categories of practitioners exercised by community health boards. If this type of health service assured more equitable and rational distribution of care, what should the position of nursing be, particularly if public participation threatened to democratize health services to the point of eliminating distinctions between professions, or if the public were more interested in warm and personalized care such as auxiliary nursing persons sometimes supply than in the theoretical and technical mastery that the professional nurse exercises?

Nursing and Undervalued Minorities:
The Example of the Elderly

When a nursing class addresses the topic of midlife crisis, students almost unanimously express a reluctance to contemplate middle age because it is the prelude to aging, and aging seems to them little better than dying. Their attitude simply reflects the prevalent social negativity toward aging and it is not likely to change as a function of nursing education. Studies suggest that nursing students' stereotypic attitudes toward the aged are changed, if at all, only by prolonged contact with elderly patients. The issue of how to change attitudes is, of course, the concern of educational psychology. The humanities must address the more fundamental issue: What images and ideals of the aged *should* health professionals be educated to have, in place of the negative stereotype of deterioration and decay? Are there more positive and freeing, and thus more human, meanings of aging that nursing and the humanities together can propose as alternatives to the concept of aging as a disease for which the cause and the cure are fervently sought?

The issue of more human meanings of aging is one for which nursing and the humanities are ideally suited to integrate their particular approaches to human experience. Historical studies are needed as a basis for understanding alternative attitudes of other cultures toward aging, as well as the origins of present values—and disvalues—of aging in this society. Against that background, an integration of the philosophical and esthetic approaches can provide an interweaving of conceptual ideals and concrete images that express the positive meanings of aging as a human value. To this fabric of meanings that the humanities weave, the nurse brings experimental meanings of aging that evolve from sustained, intimate care of the aged. The elderly, who as individuals defy generalization, often succeed where educational strategies fail to humanize the stereotypic attitudes of young professionals. Presumably, education fails where the aging themselves succeed because the latter not only present but also embody the human meanings of their experience. Education, at best, tries to neutralize negative values without offering vital, compelling alternatives. It is certain that the humanities and nursing working together can articulate such alternatives.

These then are the four categories of relation within which humanistic issues in nursing can be delineated: the nurse and the patient, the nurse and other providers, the nurse and the profession itself, and the nurse and the community. But the elucidation of all of these, using the full complement of humanities disciplines, is an ambitious program, far exceeding the scope of this volume or the project from which it derives. In the essays included here, certain relations, notably those between nurse and patient, receive greater attention than others. Moreover, all of the humanities approaches have not been utilized equally—the philosophical clearly predominates. A volume opening dialogue between nursing and the humanities is best organized around broader themes than the precise categories which more extensive inquiry, it is hoped, will elaborate. For this reason, the chapters included here have been divided on the basis of two fundamental forms of inquiry, descriptive and normative. Recognizing the distortion in any separation of "fact" and "value," we can nevertheless distinguish between those chapters in the first half of the book that portray nursing "as it is," and those in the second half that envision nursing as the authors believe it "ought to be." Thus, the two sections of the book present images and ideals of nursing, with the realization that both images and ideals may derive as much from the "eye of the beholder" as from nursing itself. But it is, after all, just that tension (often expressed during the project as the disparity between "the real and the ideal") that must enliven such discussion if it be true dialogue, an interchange which illuminates issues through the deliberate application of distinct and equally valued approaches.

Sally Gadow

Part I

IMAGES OF NURSING: CULTURAL FOUNDATIONS OF NURSING PRACTICE

Precedents and Prospects for the Humanities in Nursing*

Kathleen M. Sward

An overview of the relation between nursing and the humanities can be guided by three questions: What does the past tell us about nursing's interest in the humanities? What are the parameters that promise to shape the future of the relationship between nursing and the humanities? What is the potential now apparent for humanistic approaches in nursing education, practice, and research? It is by addressing these questions that I hope to frame a historical context for the essays that follow.

PRECEDENTS

In any discussion of modern nursing, the figure of Florence Nightingale and her activities in the last half of the 19th century and the early part of the 20th century would loom large. Certainly, they are particularly

*This paper was originally presented in response to Professor Frederick D. Kershner's "Nursing and the Humanities: Precedents, Parameters and Potential," a paper presented at a conference on "Nursing and the Humanities: A Public Dialogue," held at the University of Connecticut Health Center, Farmington, November, 1977.

appropriate to any discussion of nursing and the humanities both because of the qualities of the woman herself and because of the humanistic system of nursing she sought to establish.

Florence Nightingale was a highly intelligent upper-class woman, well educated for her time in the classical tradition. Her course of instruction from private tutors was heavily oriented toward the humanities, including grammar and composition, Greek and Latin, modern languages, music, and the history of several countries as well as constitutional history. Later, she also became well versed in the more scientific pursuits of administration, logistics, sanitation, public health, nutrition and statistics.[1] In some quarters she is known as the "Mother of Statistics." Barritt notes that literature has recognized her not just as the lady with the lamp but as the lady with the brain, "...one of those rare personalities who reshape the contours of life."[2] In 1907, she became the first, and except for one other since then, the only woman to receive the Order of Merit, given for intellectual prowess.

The many abilities of Florence Nightingale were well demonstrated when she led a group of thirty-eight nurses to care for sick, wounded, and neglected soldiers during the Crimean War. The new system of nursing she established in London in 1860 was shaped by and benefited from her background, intelligence, sensibilities, and strong humanitarian instincts. Among the innovations that she brought to her school of nursing were financial and administrative independence that enabled her to design a curriculum attentive to educational needs, independent of the immediate needs of the hospital with which the school was associated. To replace the untrained "nurses" of the time, who often included convicts and prostitutes, the school was intended to appeal to "ladies" of the middle and upper class and to others who possessed intelligence and maturity. Among other characteristics, students had to demonstrate evidence of "culture" upon entrance, presumably including some knowledge of the humanities.[3]

In modern times, the curriculum could be called patient-centered: it focused on the nursing of the sick, not the sickness; on people, not diseases. The needs of the student were also recognized with provision of time in the program for personal growth and development. This humanistic approach was not surprising in a woman who, quite literally, viewed nursing as an art.

> Nursing is an art, and if it is to be made an art, requires as exclusive a devotion, as hard a preparation as any painter's or sculptor's work, for what is having to do with dead canvas, or cold marble, compared with having to do with the living body—the temple of God's Spirit. . . . It is one of the fine arts. I had almost said, the finest of the fine arts.[4]

The history of modern nursing in this country began just over a century ago, when the first Nightingale-type schools were established in 1873. Their purpose has been viewed by some as a concern less with education than with proving that skilled nurses were better than unskilled.[5] When the demonstration was successful, hospitals everywhere sought to establish their own schools as a cheap source of skilled labor. The emphasis was on learning by doing, and Florence Nightingale's broader intent was all but lost.

Student nurses provided the bulk of bedside nursing in hospitals for many years, and even in the late 1920s 73 percent of hospitals were estimated to employ no graduate nurses in general staff positions.[6] This lack of interest in the graduate, more qualified than the student, as a provider of health care has its counterpart today. It is found in the failure of many employing institutions to value the difference in preparation between the graduate of a hospital school and the one who has had baccalaureate preparation for nursing.

However, another trend in nursing education was discernible. A program for graduate nurses in Hospital Economics was begun at Teachers College, Columbia University, in 1899. Here the first nurse professor was employed in 1906 and a Department of Nursing and Health was organized three years later. About the same time, a program that was to be a predecessor of baccalaureate programs was established as an integral part of the University of Minnesota in association with the university hospital. Five year programs combining liberal arts and nursing and leading to a Bachelor of Science degree were underway at Teachers College and Cincinnati University by 1916.[7]

The inclusion of a liberal arts component in professional preparation resulted from the long-expressed concerns of nursing educators. However, a 1959 study, Liberal Education and Nursing, revealed that concern had not been effectively matched by action: baccalaureate programs of the time were found to be greatly deficient in the liberal arts.[8] A later study identified four major factors that impeded optimum utilization of general education objectives: (1) belief that professional objectives should dominate and determine the total curriculum in a professional school; (2) confusion about the nature and purposes of general education in a nursing curriculum; (3) the discomfort of many nurse educators about education for its own sake, since it took time from nursing service needs; and, (4) a lack of leadership by nursing and college administration for the early collegiate programs in failing to insist on the primacy of the goals of liberal education.[9]

Basic nursing education programs are presently offered in hospital schools, the numbers of which are rapidly declining, and in associate and baccalaureate degree programs, which are increasing. These trends suggest that the precedents of the past, despite the odds, have fostered a lasting link between nursing and the humanities. It is the collegiate setting, where the highest percentage of educational programs for nurses are now found, that offers the greatest stimulus and opportunity for the inclusion of the humanities in the curriculum. While there is concern on some campuses about the "professionalization" of liberal arts institutions with the influx of many types of professional schools, there are also indications at other universities that the humanities as well as the professions will benefit from this movement. At a symposium on the state of the humanities held several years ago, the experience of one nationally known university was that ". . . the strongest interest in the examination, revival, and reinvigoration of the humanities has come from the professional schools."[10] Among the things that the schools seek are assistance in dealing with value questions encountered in research and practice and help with special communication needs.

PARAMETERS

From the nursing perspective, one of the parameters underlying past precedents and qualifying as a prime determiner of the future relationship between nursing and the humanities is feminism. Nurses are becoming increasingly aware of their rights and responsibilities as persons in society and are increasingly able to resist being pressured into a "woman's role" in their personal and professional lives. Sexism has been called the most pervasive problem in nursing, particularly in its relationship with the medical profession.[11] Nurses and physicians appear to be working toward collaborative roles in health care in which relationships are determined by preparation, competence, and patient needs rather than by gender. But many old stereotypes will have to be vanquished and many adjustments made before this can be accomplished. The insights provided by history, literature, and philosophy can have a prominent function in bringing this about.

What are other parameters that are crucial for shaping the future relationship between nursing and the humanities? Bulger, in his essay "Some Humanistic Issues in the Health Professions," discusses issues that focus on the relevance of the humanities for health care.[12] It may well be in the increasing interest and involvement of health professionals with these issues that the parameters of tomorrow's relationship will be most clearly developed. The issues may be grouped into four categories:

Need to Humanize Health Care

Technology and science dominate the health-care scene and are considered vital to quality health care. Still, with technology in place and scientific measures having proved their worth, results do not satisfy. The fault is not necessarily with technology or science, per se, but with the fact that these are not balanced with sensitivity and responsiveness to human need.

There is a rising chorus from both the public and professionals concerning the need to insure that health-care systems consider the humanness of those they serve. The inclusion of the humanities as a vital ingredient of professional curricula is seen as one essential means for bringing this about. The public demand is forcefully illustrated in an objection attributed to Ernest Hemingway about psychiatric treatment and writers like himself, ". . . what these shock doctors don't know is about writers and such things as remorse and contrition and what they do to them. They should make all psychiatrists take a course in creative writing so they'd know about writers. . . ."[13] A nurse educator succinctly puts the case for development of the qualities of imagination, compassion, self-realization, judgment, and feelings in nurses: "...in a society of machines, in institutions of healing run by machines, the nurse has a vital part to play in preserving the human aspects of patient care."[14] This need to humanize a technocracy in a technocratic society is seen by many as the overriding issue in health care and a challenge not only to the health care system but to 20th-century America and, perhaps, to all of modern western civilization. Bulger questions whether there can be hope for the rest of society if success is not achieved in the serving, caring professions.

Concern for the Quality of Life

There is an awareness of growing cultural boredom and anomie coupled with recognition that general social, economic, and environmental factors may have a greater impact on health than the traditional care available to the sick. This raises questions about whether illness has been defined too narrowly in contemporary society and how educational experiences for health professionals can be changed to provide the humanistic understandings increasingly necessary for effective health care.

Ethical Issues in Health Care

For health professionals, these are primarily the "bedside issues," the everyday issues of practice and research; larger ethical-legal issues such as abortion will be decided at the societal level, as will the broad political, economic, and organizational issues of health care policy.

Desire for Personal Growth

Many persons today are looking for assistance in their quest for personal meaning, particularly in the human encounters of professional practice. Bulger notes that today's students are more attuned to the affective dimensions of life than their predecessors and perhaps are more open to the insights that the humanities can contribute.

To Bulger's inventory of issues that serve so well as parameters for the future, I would add these areas in which the humanities can contribute significantly to the tasks of nursing:

The Changing Roles and Relationships Among Health Professionals and Between Health Professionals and Consumers. This is closely related to the issue of feminism but does have other origins. No longer is the physician automatically viewed as the captain of the team and the source of all information about patients' needs. There are well over 200 categories of health workers, and a number of them increasingly view themselves as professionals whose education and expertise enable them to make judgments and decisions in a specific area of health care. Medical care is an aspect of health care, but so are nursing care, special therapies, and others. The confusion in terminology which so long equated health care with medical care is slowly giving way. There is need for the humanities to relate to these changes and for the professions to recognize the assistance that might be provided by humanistic perspectives in coping with altered role perceptions and role strain.

Changing Roles and Relationships in Society at Large. The traditional family grouping is now rarer than the nontraditional. Many children may have one parent or several, teenage pregnancy is becoming a major health and social reality, and about half of all women have moved into the work force. Changes such as these have come about so fast that many health professionals have difficulty adjusting to the new life styles and sorting out their own values and feelings. The provision of needed assistance to patients could be seriously affected unless new sensitivities and ways of viewing are fostered.

The Need for Synthesis of the Humanistic and Scientific in Health Care. Novak speaks of a need for a new kind of intelligence that would differ from the rigor and quantification associated with medical and scientific knowledge but also would be unlike traditional humanistic intelligence. He believes that it should be subjective, stemming from changes in consciousness and ways of perceiving; self-critical, inventive, and alert to alternatives; and wide-ranging in order to grapple with diverse practical dilemmas. Neither medical, humanistic, professional, but related to all of these, he calls it "intelligent subjectivity."[15]

There are four skills delineated for intelligent subjectivity, ". . . the effective awareness of one's own limited personal history; an openess to noticing that of others; an effective discernment of 'sense of reality' different from one's own; and, finally, an effective awareness of those culturally derived symbolic structures of one's own perception and imagination which determine the shape of human experience."[16] These would help nurses to perceive how imagination structures experience and makes more apparent the cultural, ethical, and intellectual differences inherent in ethical dilemmas. Intelligent subjectivity could prove to be a significant, unifying, and sensitizing force in opening awareness to values central to the humanities and to the fundamental human experiences of health care.

POTENTIAL

Are there already indicators of a closer association between the humanities and nursing in the years ahead? I believe there are. Like others in society, nurses are seeking a greater measure of self-development and understanding. They are concerned about the quality of life for themselves and their patients, about their changing roles and relationships, and about the ever more difficult issues of health care. Perhaps most of all they are concerned about the need to humanize the health-care system.

Humanists, too, appear to be increasingly aware that nursing offers an extraordinary means for the practical application of the values, insights, and creativity fostered by the humanities. Jameton, writing recently in the Hastings Center Report, concluded that the nurse, not the physician, is the central figure in health care and that "Besides being philosophically important, the ethical problems of nursing are fundamental to understanding the broad ethical issues of health care institutions."[17]

Examples of the potential for a closer nursing-humanities relationship are apparent in some of the theories and directions of nursing education, nursing practice, and nursing research. An example or two in each area will serve to illustrate this.

Nursing Education

Nursing, like medicine, is considered an art and a science. Levine contends that these two aspects of the practice of the profession have been unevenly acknowledged and explored. The scientific content of patient care has been systematically developed and technological skills for the delivery of care sharpened, but the artistic use of knowledge remains only narrowly described. It is by means of the strong intellectual base provided by a liberal arts education that she believes the art and science of nursing practice will be united in the truly creative acts of human interaction and communication that result in a useful exchange between patient and nurse.[18]

Some appear to value the humanities mainly for their contribution to patient care, citing the fact that the ability to make responsible judgments in nursing requires an understanding of the patient with all the doubts, fears, fantasies, and hopes that are experienced by all human beings.[19] Wilson suggests, however, that the unique contribution of nursing to health care may lie in the utilization of scientific knowledge without destroying human rhythms, including those of the nurse. She acknowledges that there are no scientific findings linking the study of the humanities to the personal qualities of the nurse or linking the presence of qualities related to the goals of the humanities with desirable patient care. However, she maintains that the nurturing and development of the personal, human self of the nurse is the critical dimension for nursing practice. It is her belief that in addition to the expected nursing curriculum, the nurse needs ". . . an opportunity to confront and develop awareness of her own value system; an ability to separate herself, her values, and her experiences from those of others; and, a means of accepting, allowing, and integrating the different values and behaviors of others within herself."[20]

There are no voices raised against the inclusion of the humanities in the nursing curriculum. The professional accrediting body expects their inclusion and nursing educators espouse it. The real issue, it has been pointed out, is not whether they will be included but how they will be used to benefit nurses as persons and the patients in their care.[21]

Nursing Practice

The developing theory of humanistic nursing practice advanced by Paterson and Zderad views the nurse-patient relationship as one that is responsible, searching, transactional, and founded on the nurse's existential awareness of self and the other. These authors not only explore the uses of the humanities by nursing but also consider whether nursing itself is an art.

One use seen for the humanities in nursing is to broaden understanding of the human situation. In addition to their humanizing effect and their ability to stimulate imaginative creativity, the humanities are valued as a necessary complement to the heavy scientific weighting of the curriculum. Science is seen as aiming at universals, quantification, and replicability, while the arts reveal the uniqueness of the individual and are more concerned with quality, freedom, and style. Change is promoted by science, while the classics provide a sense of the unchanging and the lasting; and, although science provides the knowledge upon which decisions are based, the humanities foster examination of the values underlying practice. Thus, humanistic nursing practice is concluded to require both scientific and artistic dimensions. Each dimension has a particular purpose and each is viewed as a form of living dialogue between individuals and their human situation.[22]

The provision of a medium for the expression of nursing experience is another use considered for the humanities. Poetry is cited as an example of the interrelatedness of humanistic nursing and art. Noted are Trautman's observations that the quantity of published poems by nurses has progressively increased since the 1940s and that there has been considerable improvement in quality over the past fifteen years. This is believed due to several things: a change in nursing practice in which contemporary nursing requires more abstract thinking; increased emphasis in nursing on communication and verbal skills; and the fact that while some aspects of nursing lend themselves to scientific expression, others, equally important, can be revealed only through art. Both forms of expression contribute to clinical wisdom.[23]

Finally, the humanities are seen as useful to nursing for their therapeutic effect. The arts have long been used in nursing for this purpose, particularly with psychiatric, geriatric, and pediatric patients. "Music, poetry, painting, drama, and dance have been used effectively in various nursing situations. . . . A major therapeutic value of art lies in the fact that it confronts one with reality. . . ."[24] Through use of the various art forms, patients are helped to experience, become aware of, and express feelings.

Nursing itself as art is explored by Paterson and Zderad in terms of artful application—the response to human needs through nursing actions that are purposeful and esthetic; as useful art or a skillful doing rather than a making of a tangible product; and, finally, as a performing art. In the last, Nightingale's concept of nursing as art is echoed in a comparison made by Fahy, a nurse-educator-actress, between the process of nursing and acting in a drama:

> In a play, the actors know certain things, there are a certain number of given circumstances: plot, events, epoch, time, and plan of action, conditions of life, director's interpretation. The technical things are also there: setting, props, lights, sound effects, and so forth. But it remains at the time of curtain for the actors to go on alone and produce. In the art of nursing there are some known facts that the nursing student or the nurse can pick up: name, age, religion, ethnic background, medical diagnosis, and plan of care (sometimes), her own background knowledge and experience, and her own unique personality. However, when she encounters other patients—watch it! The same thing happens in the teaching-learning process.[25]

Paterson and Zderad contend that both art and nursing are a kind of lived dialogue, that ". . . humanistic nursing is itself an art—a clinical art—creative and existential. . . more complex than the arts of painting and poetry, for example. . . it involves being with and doing with. For the patient must participate as an active subject to actualize the possibility (form) within himself."[26]

Nursing Research

The interrelationships and implications for nursing research of philosophy, science, and theory have been examined by Silva. She questions the traditional, singular approach to the derivation of nursing knowledge which recognizes only strict adherence to the scientific method. The valuing of truths arrived at by introspection are advocated as much as those arrived at by scientific experimentation. Her premises are that all nursing theory and research are ultimately derived from or lead to philosophy, that philosophical introspection and intuition are legitimate methods of scientific inquiry, and that nursing knowledge arrived at by the scientific method too often sacrifices meaningfulness for rigor.

Silva presents evidence that knowledge derived from either the scientific or introspective methods may be correct or incorrect and that neither method leads unerringly to sound conclusions. A more holistic and less traditional approach to nursing research might therefore lead to more meaningful results.[27]

SUMMARY

Nursing education, practice, and research appear to be increasingly cognizant of and responsive to implications of nursing as both art and science. Yesterday's precedents upon which modern nursing was founded, and today's major societal concerns about health care and health professionals, support an increasing emphasis on the development of values, judgment, and compassion that complement the development of scientific knowledge and technical skills. The potential for a new and wide-ranging relationship between nursing and the humanities has perhaps never been greater. The opportunity must be seized by both, for they share a common purpose in assisting individuals toward self-understanding and creativity.

NOTES

1. Evelyn Barritt, "Florence Nightingale's Values and Modern Nursing Education," *Nursing Forum*, 12:1:11, 1973.

2. *Ibid.*, p. 9.

3. *Ibid.*, p. 26.

4. *Ibid.*, p. 25.

5. Joellen Watson, "The Evolution of Nursing Education in the United States: 100 Years of a Profession for Women," *Journal of Nursing Education*, 16:34, September, 1977.

6. Beatrice and Philip Kalisch, "Slaves, Servants, or Saints? An Analysis of the System of Nurse Training in the United States, 1873-1948," *Nursing Forum*, 14:3:226, 1975.

7. Watson, *op. cit., p. 35.*

8. Charles Russell, *Liberal Education in Nursing*, New York: Teachers College Press, Columbia University, 1959, pp. 116-117.

9. Mary Pillepich, *Development of General Education in Collegiate Nursing Programs: Role of the Administrator*, New York: Teachers College Press, Columbia University, 1962, pp. 58-65.

10. "A Symposium on the State of the Humanities," *Change Magazine*, Special Issue on the Future of the Humanities, 7:43, Summer, 1975.

11. Virginia Cleland, "Sex Discrimination: Nursing's Most Pervasive Problem," *American Journal of Nursing*, 71:1542-1547, August, 1971.

12. Roger Bulger, "Some Humanistic Issues in the Health Professions," *Health Care Dimensions: Health Care Issues*, (ed.) Madeline Leininger, Philadelphia: F.A. Davis Company, 1974, pp. 29-36.

13. Fitzhugh Mullan, "Asylum from Asylums," *New York Times Book Review*, February 5, 1978, p. 31.

14. Holly Wilson, "A Case for Humanities in Professional Nursing Education," *Nursing Forum*, 13:4:414, 1974.

15. Michael Novak, "The Liberation of Imagination: The Place of Intelligent Subjectivity in Health Care Education," *Man and Medicine*, 1:95-107, Winter, 1976.

16. *Ibid.*, p. 104.

17. Andrew Jameton, "The Nurse: When Roles and Rules Conflict," *Hastings Center Report*, 7:22, August, 1977.

18. Myra Levine, "On Creativity in Nursing," *Image*, 5:3:15-19, 1973.

19. Charles Berry and E.J. Drummond, "The Place of the Humanities in Nursing Education," *Nursing Outlook*, 18:30-31, September, 1970.

20. Wilson, *op. cit.*, p. 415.

21. Mark and Carole Siegel, "The Use of Literature in Professional Nursing Education," *Nursing Forum*, 16:2:158, 1977.

22. Josephine Paterson and Loretta Zderad, *Humanistic Nursing*, New York: John Wiley and Sons, 1976, pp. 95-97.

23. *Ibid.*, pp. 95-96, citing Mary Jane Trautman, "Nurses as Poets," *American Journal of Nursing*, 71:727-728, April, 1971.

24. *Ibid.*, p. 97.

25. *Ibid.*, pp. 99-100, citing Ellen Fahy, "Nursing Process as a Performing Art," *Humanities and the Arts as Bases for Nursing*, Lennox, Mass.: New England Council on Higher Education for Nursing, June, 1968, p. 124.

26. Paterson and Zderad, *op. cit.*, p. 101.

27. Mary Silva, "Philosophy, Science, Theory: Interrelationships and Implications for Nursing Research," *Image*, 9:59-63, October, 1977.

BIBLIOGRAPHY

Barritt, Evelyn. "Florence Nightingale's Values and Modern Nursing Education," *Nursing Forum*, 12:1:7-47, 1973.

Berry, Charles and E.J. Drummond. "The Place of the Humanities in Nursing Education," *Nursing Outlook*, 18:30-31, September, 1973.

Bulger, Roger. "Some Humanistic Issues in the Health Professions," *Health Care Dimensions: Health Care Issues*, (ed.) Madeline Leininger, Philadelphia: F. A. Davis Company, 1974.

Cleland, Virginia. "Sex Discrimination: Nursing's Most Pervasive Problem," *American Journal of Nursing*, 71:1542-1547, August, 1971.

Jameton, Andrew. "The Nurse: When Roles and Rules Conflict," *Hastings Center Report*, 7:22-23, August, 1977.

Kalish, Beatrice and Philip. "Slaves, Servants, or Saints? An Analysis of the System of Nurse Training in the United States, 1873-1948," *Nursing Forum*, 14:3:223-263, 1975.

Levine, Myra. "On Creativity in Nursing," *Image*, 5:3:15-19, 1973.

Mullan, Fitzhugh. "Asylum From Asylums," *New York Times Book Review*, February 5, 1978, pp. 13, 30-31.

Novak, Michael. "The Liberation of Imagination: The Place of Intelligent Subjectivity in Health Care Education," *Man and Medicine*, 1:95-107, Winter, 1976.

Paterson, Josephine and Loretta Zderad. *Humanistic Nursing*. New York: John Wiley and Sons, 1976.

Pillepich, Mary. *Development of General Education in Collegiate Nursing Programs: Role of the Administrator*. New York: Teachers College Press, 1962.

Russell, Charles. *Liberal Education in Nursing*. New York: Teachers College Press, 1959.

Siegel, Mark and Carole. "The Use of Literature in Professional Nursing Education, *Nursing Forum*, 16:2:158-164, 1977.

Silva, Mary. "Philosophy, Science, Theory: Interrelationships and Implications for Nursing Research," *Image*, 9:59-63, October, 1977.

"Symposium on the State of the Humanities," *Change Magazine*, Summer, 1975.

Watson, Joellen. "The Evolution of Nursing Education in the United States: 100 Years of a Profession for Women," *Journal of Nursing Education*, 16:31-37, September, 1977.

Wilson, Holly. "A Case for Humanities in Professional Nursing Education," *Nursing Forum*, 13:4:406-417, 1974.

Images in Conflict

The Fractured Image:
The Public Stereotype
of Nursing and the Nurse

Mila Ann Aroskar

Many questions can be posed about the public image of the nurse and nursing. For example, are there single or multiple public images? In what forms do(es) the image(s) exist? Is the public image of nursing congruent with the image or images held by the nursing profession of itself? It is assumed that images are socially and culturally determined and may change in terms of time and place as people interact with their environment. Simmons, a sociologist, reminds us that the "imaged" characteristics under consideration may or may not actually exist in reality. They are perceived to exist and consequently provide pressure on the actual behavior of both the image-bearer, in this case the nurse, and his or her potential clients or patients. The significance

18

of the image lies not in its validity but in the firmness and energy with which it is held and the influence that it exerts on actual behavior.[1]

The hypothesis of this chapter is that cracks and conflicts exist in the public image of the nurse and in the profession's own image of the service it delivers to this same public or publics. For example, the *intra*disciplinary image of the nurse involved in promotion and maintenance of health in community settings does not seem to exist in the public image. A subhypothesis is that the traditional "handmaid of the physician" image still exists as a public image of the nurse. Nurses in hospitals are the major focus of this chapter because 90 percent of nurses work in hospitals even though 90 percent of patients are elsewhere in the health-care system—for example, ambulatory care settings. Additionally, the majority of nurses are still educated in hospital schools although this is changing. This change was accelerated with publication of the Position Paper in 1965 by the American Nurses' Association. The Position Paper states that the minimum level for beginning professional nursing practice should be a baccalaureate degree education. Commitment is also made to the concept that all nursing education should take place in institutions of higher education.

TESTING AND SAMPLING OPINIONS

A small informal sampling by the author doing a word association test with a few acquaintances and strangers gave some clues to the image of nurses which individuals carry around with them. Asked to give the first word they thought of when "nurse" was mentioned, respondents said: Hospital, doctor, registered, female, white uniform, and professional. Respondents were of both sexes, ranged from the teens to the seventies in age, and had such labels as lawyer, real estate agent, grandmother, and supermarket cashier. (According to Simmons these are "outsiders" to the focal group, that is, nurses. Examples of "insiders" would be persons in similar or related positions, e.g., physicians, lab technicians.[2]) The majority of responses indicate the more traditional viewpoint while a minority mentioned the "newer" image of the nurse which was promoted by Florence Nightingale more than 100 years ago. Olesen and Whittaker compare the traditional and contemporary views of nursing work. Under the traditional view one finds the following characteristics:[3]

Traditional	Contemporary
High technical skill	Originality and creativity
Emotional control and constraint	Exercise of imagination and insight
Human drama and excitement	Solid intellectual content
Clear-cut lines of authority	Frequent innovation in solution of problems
Order and routine	
Hard work	
Meticulousness	
Close supervision and direction	
Clearly defined work tasks; each person responsible for her job and her job alone	

To the list of contemporary views, the author would add that of decision-maker.

Recent research in the area of the public image of the nurse is rather skimpy and has been done with small samples. However, it provides some support for saying that the traditional view of nursing still remains and is perpetuated by the media. This is in contrast with research reported in the 1940s and early 1950s which indicated different, conflicting images of the nurse held by different social classes, public officials, physicians, nurses, and so on. These studies were conducted in the era before TV dominated much of our home entertainment, interestingly enough.[4]

An opinion poll in the 1970s of twenty-five citizens found that the major image presented on TV and in books is the nurse as a sex symbol or as having romantic relationships. The nurse has a subordinate role to the physician and generally lacks intelligence. Nurses are seen as having devoted hearts and disciplined hands but not necessarily inquiring minds. Yet the majority of respondents in this survey while equating nursing with the female sex felt the media image was inaccurate. Some said they had gone to a physician for treatment or advice which could have been provided by a nurse and felt that nurses could act independently of physicians. However, none of the respondents mentioned the more cognitive roles that nurses have as researchers, teachers, administrators, planners, or providers of primary care.[5] These findings are in direct contrast with an informal sampling done by Pender in the New Haven area among nonmedical acquaintances.

In another study reported in 1976, Beletz found that a small sample of hospitalized patients identified activities of the nurse which had many commonalities with the image projected on TV programs. Taking doctors' orders, giving medications, serving meals, giving shots, and providing bedpans were mentioned as nursing activities by the respondents. Nurses were seen as having limited functions in the larger community outside the hospital. When asked if nurses should visit people after discharge from the hospital to answer questions and check progress, responses were: "if a doctor recommended a nurse"; "only a doctor should do this"; "it would be a waste of a resource and of the nurses' time"; "for elderly people or children"; "okay for the lower socioeconomic levels"; "I doubt if it's needed with private cases, and would probably be resisted."[6] The investigator concluded that nurses in this general hospital where the study was conducted were apparently not practicing according to a professional model and that patients had little knowledge of what nurses could do within and outside of hospital walls.[7]

In a study of high school senior boys' attitudes toward nursing as a career, the investigator found that nursing is seen as the occupation of lowest masculinity when compared with other occupations such as architectural engineer, social worker, pharmacist, chemist, school counselor, and teacher.[8] This reinforces the notion that nursing is women's work even though historically nursing has been done by men since the Crusades in both the religious and the secular contexts. Even in the United States a large percentage of nursing services was performed by men in the early part of the 19th century. Yet the predominant labels for those who care for the sick in Western culture are profoundly female—for example, "sister" as applied not only to religious functionaries but also the nurse. Additionally, "nursing" implies a mother's relationship to her children, caring for her family and managing her home, with no formal boundaries to her area of competence. These are the images which still link nursing so strongly with the female role.[9]

MEDIA IMAGES

Television and movies continue to reinforce this female image of the nurse. The image presented is someone who can work everywhere without specialized training for different roles. This generally happens because the nurse is a contract player used simply for purposes of the story. Nurses are also represented as busy, rarely seen with patients, or making independent decisions. They act like medical secretaries, put flowers in vases, answer telephones, or are coldly efficient like Nurse Ratched in "One Flew Over the Cuckoo's Nest."[10] These portrayals of nursing perpetuate traditional stereotypes and fail to inform the public of what nursing can and should be providing in terms of nursing services, e.g., nurse practitioners in joint practices in ambulatory care.

Wheelock, a professor of English, discusses the film image of nurses as sex objects in pornographic films. He compares nurses, teachers, and stewardesses in hypothesizing that there are excellent opportunities for sexual fantasizing in a hierarchical social structure which maintains men at the top and women as subject to the orders and decisions made by these men. He states that pornographic films transform nurses and stewardesses into an "American geisha class" where women are no threat and do everything they are told to do by men. His evidence is drawn from films of the 1950s, "Not as a Stranger" and "The Blob" and "M.A.S.H." in 1970. These films play on the themes of obedience to higher authority and the assumption that nurses are dumb because they obey this authority. Since nurses talk about "total patient care" and have extensive knowledge of and exposure to the human body this may provoke expectations related to meeting of sexual needs.[11] In looking at the physician-nurse relationship, the sexual cannot be overlooked whether it is myth or reality. According to Mauksch, the "definition of the nurse as a sexual target is one of the most severe obstacles to colleague-like, professional, and intellectual relations."[12]

In summary, the media, the practice of nursing in bureaucratic institutions, and lack of public knowledge about the activities involved in professional nursing practice contribute to the traditional image of the nurse as a female lacking in initiative and intelligence who is obedient to the authority of the physician. It is difficult from the above bits of research and media articles to gain any generalized notion of the realistic image, the reflected, or the ideal image of nursing held by the profession and the public.

However, the above samples do indicate cracks in today's image which will be discussed further in this chapter. I would like to look first at some of the historical, socioeconomic, and educational factors which explain in part how this image of the nurse presented above has been perpetuated in the United States into the 1970s.

HISTORICAL, SOCIOECONOMIC, AND EDUCATIONAL CONTEXT

Over 100 years ago, Florence Nightingale, a member of the English upper class, had a startling insight for the time—that one needed to *learn* how to be a nurse. In the middle of the 19th century it was universally assumed that the only qualification for taking care of the sick was to be a woman. Family nursing experiences made Nightingale realize that knowledge and expert skill were necessary to bring relief to the sick.[13]

In 1845, hospitals were places of squalor and degradation. Both patients and nurses suffered from the intolerable conditions of filth. Hospital nurses were known to be drunkards who were notoriously immoral.[14] However, Nightingale was determined to train as a nurse and then to reform nursing by producing "a new type of nurse"—a respectable, reliable, and qualified individual.[15] Difficulties in preparing this nurse continued because of the public image of the nurse as a "self-immolating sister of charity." Few could visualize the professional nurse, trained, efficient, and highly paid which Nightingale projected for women of any class.[16] At the Nightingale School the two goals of training and education of this type of nurse were the acquisition of knowledge and the development of character.[17] These paradoxical

strands, secular and religious, moral and immoral, educated and uneducated, still meet today in education and practice for individuals
and the profession, and inevitably, in the public image of the nurse.

It should be noted in view of nursing's continuing struggle to become more independent from medicine, that when Nightingale went
to Turkey to provide nursing service in the military hospitals her
authority sanctioned by the English government for everything related
to nursing was "... subject of course to the sanction and approval of
the chief medical officer."[18] Nursing care was viewed as an essential
service but as subservient to medical care. This was a battle that
Nightingale never did win.

Most of the discussion in this next section comes from Ashley's Doctoral dissertation reported in the book *Hospitals, Paternalism, and the
Role of the Nurse*. In the United States, the development of modern
nursing and nursing education must be viewed in the context of the
development of hospitals as a social institution where major concerns
are about business efficiency rather than humanitarianism.[19]

The need for development of schools of nursing became evident in
the United States in the late 1800s after the resulting improvement in
patient care in England where trained nurses were introduced into the
hospital system. Unfortunately the schools were not financially independent as were the Nightingale Schools in England. Instead, an apprenticeship arrangement was established. The school agreed to give
nursing service to the hospitals in exchange for the hospitals' provision
of clinical experience for students. Establishing a school of nursing
became accepted as the most popular and least expensive way of providing nursing care,[20] often the major service offered by hospitals to
patients.

Nursing education thus remained entirely dependent on the kind
and quality of medical services provided in the hospitals for teaching
purposes. Education of nurses was not a hospital priority. There was
no Flexner Report to point out the inadequate, inhumane conditions
under which nursing students labored or to warn the public that the
source of most hospital nursing care was students who worked from
60 to 105 hours per week.[21]

A paternalistic, laissez-faire approach, a philosophy of individual-
ism for hospital administrators and physicians, and structured in-

equality within hospitals impeded any attempts to change hospital organization and the delivery of nursing care. As late as the 1930s many hospitals employed no paid instructors and provided little formal instruction for students.[22] Does one detect a note of anti-intellectualism in nursing here? Where is recognition of Nightingale's contention that nursing must be learned? As early as 1896, Mary Adelaide Nutting was one of the first nursing leaders to express public concern about the abuse of students by so-called "schools" and hospitals. Yet, the practice of using nursing students as the main nursing staff of the hospital continued to the 1950s and beyond. This is one of the reasons why hospital costs were kept artificially low for decades.[23]

The only criterion applied by hospitals as businesses was the economic one. The humanitarian motive was submerged in the economic. Unfortunately, nursing provided a major support for continuance of this criterion when members of the nurses' Society of Superintendents were asked to participate in the work of the American Hospital Association's Committee on Training Schools in the first decade of the 20th century.[24] In the 1920s the superintendents became associate members of the A.H.A. At this level of membership they had no voting power and no influence on the organization's policies. Also in the hospital hierarchy, the superintendents were in a subservient position to hospital administrators and boards of trustees. These women were responsible both for students (the school) and care of patients (the hospital). Needs of students were generally subordinated to those of the hospital because of the apprenticeship arrangement. There was no innovation or change unless it was approved by the superiors, that is, physicians and hospital administrators.[25] Becoming nonvoting members of the A.H.A. did not advance the cause of education of students or change the subservient position of nurses in the male-dominated hierarchy.

When the first nursing schools were established in the United States, the family was the institutional model for the operation of hospitals. All policies and procedures were designed to guide the management of the "household":

The role of women (nurses) was very early conceived as that of caring for the "hospital family." Their purpose was to provide efficient, economical production in the form of patient care; they were to be loyal to the institution and devoted to preserving its reputation. Through service and self-sacrifice, they were to work continuously to keep the "family" happy. All the departments of the hospital—from wards and operating rooms to storerooms and kitchens—depended upon the continuous presence of nurses. For 24 hours a day, nurses were expected to be versatile in their skills, to demonstrate their ability to take care of whatever needs night arise, whether in the area of patient care, medical treatment, housekeeping, dispensing drugs, or supervising the diet and the kitchen. Like mothers in a household, nurses were responsible for meeting the needs of all members of the hospital family—from patients to physicians. Continuous responsibility for the care of those confined to hospital beds is still the unique function of the nursing profession.

In addition, women (nurses) were expected to look out for the needs of men (the physicians) in the hospital family, who, for the most part, did not reside in the household, but were free to come and go. In the absence of men, women were expected to assume full responsibility for their decision-making functions by taking on the male role themselves. This decision-making role was, of course, relinquished upon the return of the men. Nurses were, and still are, constantly supportive of the institution, especially of its male members, and constantly busy.[26]

This very long quote was included here because it includes so many aspects of the family model which is still perpetuated in many hospitals—mother, father, and kids (patients). Physicians provide support for the "household" by bringing in patients. Nurses function as "homemakers." This model was evident at two large medical centers with which I was associated as student and staff member in the early 1960s. It is a model embedded as well in the cultural configuration of our society.

Essentially the same picture emerged in a 1968 book by Duff and Hollingshead, *Sickness and Society*. Nursing roles in the bureaucracy were complex and filled with contradictions as described in the above quotation.[27] Nurses were expected to carry out the physician's orders as a "personal assistant" to the physician. Patients indicated that they expected the nurse to make only minor decisions concerning their care while physicians made the major decisions. Nurses also accepted this role of the physician as the legally and professionally responsible primary decision-maker. Patients, families, and nurses merely complied with the physician's decisions. The conclusion of the Duff and Hollingshead work was that physicians and patients did not want the nurse's role to be anything more than a relatively passive one—providing technical services in an atmosphere of "tender loving care"![28]

The emphasis on obedience in nursing in the Victorian era is revealed in another statement of directives for hospital nurses:

> In addition to caring for your 50 patients, each nurse will follow these regulations:...Daily sweep and mop the floors of your ward, dust the patient's furniture and window sills...The nurse's notes are important in aiding the physician's work. Make your pens carefully; you may whittle nibs to your individual taste...Graduate nurses in good standing with the director of nurses will be given an evening off each week for courting purposes or two evenings a week if you go regularly to church...Any nurse who smokes, uses liquor in any form, gets her hair done at a beauty shop, or frequents dance halls will give the director of nurses good reason to suspect her worth, intentions and integrity.[29]

Such directives may account for the upper-class image of the nurse as a domestic servant and the middle-class image that nursing was good training for a wife to have although it was more desirable for middle-class daughters to go to college where they could meet "people in their own class." The lower class viewed nursing "...one of the noblest of all professions" and felt that the nurse's knowledge would be advantageous as both a wife and mother.[30]

While nursing has moved away from such strict emphasis on obedience, it is still considered to be a desirable attribute of nurses. A study conducted in the 1960s concluded that the predominant atmosphere in nursing schools was authoritarian.[31] Profiles of nursing students in the late 1960s showed some tendency to be submissive, to sustain a subordinate role, and to have stronger needs for deference and self-abasement than non-nursing students.[32] [33] These characteristics seem to be changing in baccalaureate nursing students but they still have the bureaucratic structure to contend with as students and practitioners.

Marlene Kramer has described in her studies of professional-bureaucratic role conflict the frustrations of new graduates who try to act creatively and independently in the bureaucracy. Nurses' actions are determined to such a large extent by prescribed routines, policies, administrative directives, and physicians' orders that there is little freedom left for the nurse to exercise professional judgment. Twenty percent of the nurses in Kramer's studies leave nursing completely. Others move from job to job seeking a situation where they can behave more independently in regard to patient care.[34] How can students develop a sense of autonomy when they see so few nurses practicing in an autonomous manner? Recall the findings of the Beletz and Duff and Hollingshead studies cited previously. Another piece of this picture is provided in the Murphy study of levels of moral reasoning in a group of staff and supervisory nurses. Most participants were at the conventional level of moral reasoning, i.e., obedient to authority, and needing harmonious relationships with institutions and authority figures.[35] These factors influence nursing behavior in a powerful way.

Nursing, perhaps more than any other profession, has been influenced by social concepts regarding the nature of women and their place in society. Legal recognition in the form of practice acts made the nurse's subservience to physicians even more evident. Unfortunately, the legal and educational systems have contributed to the repression of nurses as much as the medical-care system itself.

Many nurses have always functioned independently as professionals, but most do not because it is not legal under present laws for them to do so. Nurse practice acts give men the legal right to supervise women in a paternalistic system whether they are present or not when nursing care is delivered. Medical supervision is in most instances a myth. Nursing care goes on without either the consultation or the presence of the doctor. Absentee supervision is a reality in practice that should have legal recognition. Yet a statement by the American Medical Association's Committee on Nursing approved by the association in 1970 made the assumption that nurses will remain in their "logical place at the physician's side" functioning under the physician's supervision for the purpose of "extending the hands of the physician."[36] This statement was made at the same time that nurses in many states were struggling to change the legal basis for nursing practice on a professional model of autonomy in nurse practice acts.

Even new definitions of nursing in nurse practice acts such as that of New York State, which was heralded in 1972 as a triumph for professional nursing, still incorporate the traditional view of the nurse in the medical sphere as a dependent functionary. The nurse does not function independently in the medical sphere but must act under a physician's direction and supervision—*the myth perpetuated in the late 20th century*. There is a dichotomy between medical and nursing functions in relation to "diagnosing" and "treating" but these functions as carried out by nurses are somewhat vague in the New York definition.[37] The "extended" or "expanded" role of the nurse into traditionally medical areas of practice is not legally recognized in this definition.

The California definition manages to avoid perpetuating traditional concepts of nursing's medical role but indicates that the nurse's and physician's functions overlap to some extent and that the two professions work collaboratively in this area. The California preamble and definition indicate that the Legislature recognized the expanded role of the nurse with respect to the performance of medical acts and intended to legitimize these acts without any overriding requirement of physician delegation or supervision. However, this definition also demonstrates the difficulty of formulating redefinitions of practice which take into account the evolving role of the nurse.[38] These evolving efforts at legal redefinition of nursing can provide an important forum for the public to learn more about professional nursing and what they can expect from nurses in terms of practice.

A recent survey of fifty-seven practicing physicians in one community in the Eastern United States found that the majority of respondents saw nurses performing such extended functions as the patient's health history, triage of patients and making referrals to appropriate physicians, performing diagnostic procedures, making initial house calls to assess a patient's condition, managing child health supervision, initiating treatment in cardiac arrest, anaphylactic shock, and respiratory distress, and prescribing medications for minor symptoms, pain relief, and sedation. The physicians also indicated that the extended role should be practiced under their supervision. Supervision is not defined or discussed.[39] These extended roles are generally viewed as complementary and supplementary to physician care—not a substitute. One wonders if nurses have moved very far from the traditional "handmaid of the physician" role in taking on even these extended functions. On the other hand, these very functions may and do provide the opportunity that nurses want to practice preventive health care in other than hospital settings, which is the traditional public image of nursing practice.

Looking further at the role of women vis-à-vis men and nurses vis-à-vis doctors in our society, one considers the findings of the Broverman et al. study and Stein's perceptive writings on the doctor-nurse game. The Broverman et al. study found that male and female mental health clinicians (46 male and 33 female psychiatrists, psychologists, and social workers) have a double standard for mental health of men and women. The results were as follows:

1. There was high agreement among clinicians as to the attributes characterizing healthy adult men, healthy adult women, and healthy adults, sex unspecified.
2. There were no differences among men and women clinicians.
3. Clinicians had different standards of health for men and women. Their concepts of healthy mature men did not differ significantly from their concepts of healthy mature adults, but their concepts of healthy mature women did differ significantly from those for men and for adults. Clinicians were likely to suggest that women differ from healthy men by being more submissive, less independent, less adventurous, more easily influenced, less aggressive, less competitive, more excitable in minor crises, more easily hurt, more emotional, more conceited about their appearance, less objective, and less interested in math and science. Finally, what was judged healthy for adults, sex unspecified, and for adult males, was in general highly correlated with previous studies of social desirability as perceived by nonprofessional subjects.[40]

It seems evident that for a woman to be judged "healthy" in our society, she must adjust to and accept the behavioral norms for the female sex even though these characteristics are regarded as less socially desirable. Broverman et al. remark that "This constellation seems a most unusual way of describing any mature, healthy individual." The double standard of sexual mental health existing side by side with a single and masculine standard of *human* mental health is enforced by both society and clinicians. Women are in a double bind if they wish to act as mature adults as defined in our culture.[41]

Consider the doctor-nurse game described by Leonard Stein as a manifestation of how nurses accomplish certain goals related to patient care in their interactions with physicians. According to Stein, the physician has traditionally had total responsibility for decision-making regarding the management of the patient's treatment. The physician gathers data from several sources to make these decisions— for example, doing a thorough physical examination, interpreting laboratory findings, and, sometimes, obtaining recommendations from consultant physicians. Recommendations are also received from nurses. Stein analyzes the interaction between doctor and nurse through which these recommendations by nurses are made and received.[42]

The object of the "game," as perceived by Stein, is that the nurse should be bold, take initiative, and be responsible for making recommendations while appearing passive at the same time. This is done in such a manner as to make her recommendations appear to be initiated by the physician. There are penalties on both sides if the players fail too frequently. The most important rule of the game is that open disagreement is to be avoided at all costs by both sides. Thus nurses must communicate their recommendations without appearing to do so. Rewards from playing the game are that the doctor-nurse "team" operates efficiently. Successful game playing leads to a doctor-nurse alliance in which the nurse is used as a valuable consultant and the doctor has his path smoothed by nurses for getting his work done, e.g., charts are organized and his pet routines carefully followed.[43]

Stein says that the nurse who sees herself as a consultant but refuses to follow the rules in playing the game "has hell to pay." She is labelled as a "bitch" by doctors and is constantly reminded in several ways that she is not loved. This game evolved through the education of both physicians and nurses which shaped attitudes necessary for playing the game. The nurse learns the game from her first days in nursing school through instructors who often are ambivalent about the role of the professional nurse. Some of these instructors explicitly tell students that their femininity is an important asset to be used in relating to physicians.

Stein analyzes some of the factors that preserve this game-playing in the medical arena. He says that one of the factors is sexual roles. The majority of doctors are men and approximately 98 percent of nurses are women. The various elements of the doctor-nurse game reinforce the stereotyped roles of male dominance and female passivity. Additionally, independent action for nursing students is generally prohibited. This inhibition of independent action is most marked when relating to the physician.[44] Although no longer common practice, the author knows of hospitals where nursing students must still rise and give their seats to doctors when they come into a patient unit. This game supports and protects a rigid organizational structure with physicians remaining in clear authority. On the other hand, one also finds nurses working in more collaborative relationships, e.g., primary nursing. At the risk of sounding naive, I suggest that one hope for ridding the system of this game is through genuine interdisciplinary learning experiences where students do not have to learn this particular game.

In summary, the nurse who tries to practice as a human and humane professional in the present system is still often enmeshed in a historical, social, and cultural maze which views women primarily in a submissive role.

EVIDENCE AND HOPE FOR CHANGE

There is hope that significant change can occur within the social context of the health care system. Nurses are forming coalitions for political action in many parts of the country as well as presenting a stronger lobby on the Washington scene. One controversial media figure told the author that in her observations of the women's movement around the country, the efforts to promote better health care for and by women is without a doubt the most significant part of the movement with the most potential for meeting its goals over a period of time. This is a superb opportunity for nurses to share their knowledge and expertise with both individuals and families, if they choose to do so in formal and informal settings.

Nurses, the largest group of practitioners in the health field, may yet be able to do what philosophers Dickoff and James call "philosophic nursing," that is, action preceded and guided by thought, within a specific model of health care.[45] Such a model might incorporate the following aspects: health care is considered to be the right of each individual; is comprehensive; is available to all persons seeking it; is both individual-centered and family-centered (the individual is a participant in decision-making regarding his or her health); is provided by a team of health workers; is an integral part of community services; individual and family have the basic responsibility for meeting their needs; and health care is provided within the individual's life style to the extent wished by and allowed by her or his health state.[46] There is some evidence throughout the United States in traditional and nontraditional health care settings that pieces of this model are available in the form of nursing services for the public.[47] Nurses must continue efforts to approximate this or similar health models in services provided through individual practice and legislative efforts. Consumers can demand such services only if they know they can and do exist.

As Simmons says, reliable information on the public image of a profession can be very helpful to its leaders if they are alert enough to take positive action toward shaping public opinion in support of their special services.[48] Nurses have not taken advantage of the expertise of advertising and public relations organizations to promote the image of the *professional* nurse which can be seen in primary care settings, for example. The predominant public image of the nursing profession today reflects the traditional image of the woman as nurse. Maybe the public does not want to change this image! Yet the traditional image may become plural as the public(s) has experiences with newer models of health and nursing care, for example, joint practices where physicians and nurses work in collaborative and complementary arrangements reflecting different blends of the natural and social sciences in their educational bases.[49] Somehow, the "human side" of patient/client care must be integrated with the professional and technical aspects of practice. Nursing is making an effort to accomplish this goal even in many bureaucratic health care settings.

Perhaps, as Newton suggests in her essay in this chapter, we need new terms for the different functional roles within nursing today. The term "nurse" may be appropriate for specified persons performing certain activities which continue to be functional for certain aspects of sick patient care. On the other hand, different behaviors related to health promotion and maintenance may need different labels. A hint of this is seen in the Lysaught Report which talked about nursing in terms of episodic and distributive care. These ideas need to be explored by the profession with an open mind. There may be several images of what we now know as nursing, that is, multiple realities. Nursing may not be a "melting pot" any more than our society is. Maybe the doorway is open to legitimizing pluralism in the culture of nursing. Until then, the question "Will the real nurse please stand up?" cannot be answered.

A Vindication of the Gentle Sister: Comment on "The Fractured Image"

Lisa Newton

Dr. Aroskar presents a convincing case for the thesis that there is a terrible disparity between the public image of the nurse and the reality of the contemporary nurse. I think that her statement about the derivation of the public image from historical precedents (and historical accidents) is sound. I also believe that she is correct in her insistence that nurses, as currently trained, are capable of greatly expanded roles in a rapidly expanding system of health care, roles that presuppose an autonomous professional nurse instead of the traditional obedient "sister."

I take the general drift of her argument to be unexceptionable. Therefore, I will limit my commentary to raising a question about the assumption that lies behind Dr. Aroskar's statement—the assumption that, if the professional competence of the contemporary nurse and the public image of the nurse are at odds, there is necessarily something wrong with the public image. In other words, Dr. Aroskar assumes that the relationship between public image and contemporary nursing is necessarily *only* empirical: the image is "what the public thinks the contemporary nurse is in fact," and if the contemporary nurse is in fact different, then the public image is simply incorrect. If that is all there is to the relationship, then the remedy for the discrepancy is, as Dr. Aroskar suggests, a massive, educative public relations campaign. Nevertheless, it should be noted that the relationship need not be entirely descriptive. It may be at least in part prescriptive, setting a norm for the nurse that the public, for some reason, finds desirable. In fact, a case could be made that the traditional image, or "public stereotype," of the nurse prescribes a health-care role that is still coherent, possible, and functional. Indeed, the public may have good reasons for encouraging nurses to conform to that image for the patient's benefit, and a nurse who by inclination and training is not prepared to assume that role may do much better for herself under a different professional description. I will attempt to make that case in what follows in order to point up the importance of Dr. Aroskar's assumption, and the crucial place it holds in her argument. If this assumption is changed, a completely different set of consequences follows.

Let us consider the image of the Gentle Sister, the highly skilled but sweetly submissive nurse of tradition. This image, introduced by Dr. Aroskar, is familiar to all of us since we were all probably raised with some variant of it. This image presents a profession of "devoted hearts and disciplined hands but not necessarily inquiring minds . . . , taking doctors' orders, giving medications, serving meals, giving shots, and providing bedpans." This traditional image *is* "the Nurse" of popular culture, and for the remainder of my argument, unless otherwise stated, I shall use the term "Nurse" to refer to this traditional image. Under the doctor's supervision (in accordance with his scientific education), the Nurse *nurtures* the patient, attending to basic and intimate physical needs. Because of this nurturing, the Nurse is strongly linked to maternal images. Hence, the Nurse is necessarily female and (as the image comes full circle) justifiably subject to men (the doctors) since men are supposed to be naturally superior to women. The interface between the feminine aspect of the Nurse and the antiseptic aspect of the medical setting in which she works is subject to shift, and the image supports both the coldly efficient floor supervisor that enforces every rule, and the sweet young thing that flirts with the interns. The heart of the image is the devoted mother with the technical skill to translate devotion into healing.

The subservience of nursing practice to medical practice never required justification beyond the presumed sapiential authority of the physician. While simple sexism may have accounted for some of its less attractive aspects, its foundation was the unquestioned assumption that the physician knew what was wrong with the patient and what treatment he or she should be receiving, and that the Nurse's knowledge was limited to a knowledge of the means to implement the physician's decisions. Dr. Aroskar suggests at one point (following Wheelock) that the Nurse is subject to the physician because she is a woman (a sex object), and presumed to be less knowledgeable than he just because of that subjection. However, the reverse of that causal sequence is more plausible—the Nurse is subject to the physician (nursing practice is subject to medical practice) because of the superior knowledge of the physician, and the Nurse is free to assume traditionally female characteristics (tenderness, sympathy) and act out female subroles ("mothering," trivial scolding, protecting), precisely because these characteristics and subroles are imaged as compatible only with subservient roles. This sequence would explain why promotion to floor supervisor (e.g. Nurse Ratched in Kesey's *One Flew Over the Cuckoo's Nest*) is commonly associated with suppression of the "female" aspect of the Nurse; supervisors, as occupying a "male" role, are not "permitted" the female-imaged characteristics of gentleness and sympathy. As the physician's authority is legitimately sapiential, the Nurse's best efforts to improve the condition of the patient consist in absolute obedience to the physician's instructions. Since obedience is known to be difficult for humans, the highly disciplined settings of convent and military service, with their emphasis on the inculcation of a habit of obedience, provided the best background for Nursing.

Hence the military and religious model of nursing practice that still prevails.

Such is the image. And I would contend that there is, logically, not much wrong with it. Dr. Aroskar's claim to the contrary notwithstanding, it contains no paradoxes, contradictions, mazes, or irreconcilable conflicts, if understood simply as a definition of a role. It describes a possible role or occupation, a possible pattern of human action. As a subservient role, it holds no attraction for me, nor probably for you; but that is not the question. The question is, could it hold any attraction for any human being and are there people who could fill it? The answer to this is certainly yes. With varying degrees of willingness, nursing students and nursing sisters have filled this role for a century and more. Certainly the role would prove satisfying for those with the "tendency to be submissive, to sustain a subordinate role, and to have [strong] needs for deference and self-abasement," that some nursing students seem to have. The "prescribed routines, policies, administrative directives, and physicians' orders" that circumscribe the Nurse's life would not be a source of frustration to those inclined to and prepared for a subordinate role. We would have to agree that the Nurse, evaluated in isolation, is an undesirable human being by customary standards of normal adulthood because she lacks the responsibility and initiative which we associate with autonomous maturity. But the Nurse in context, as a subordinate role in a complex structure of authority, should not be evaluated by those standards. An autonomous human being can certainly fill a nonautonomous role if there are sufficiently good reasons to do so.

The Nurse is a coherent role (logically consistent), and a humanly possible one (human beings can fill it and even find satisfaction in it). We must now ask if it is functional in the health-care setting, i.e. does it correspond to a real and essential need. Again, there can be little doubt that it is, and does. As long as there are prescribed treatments that patients cannot administer to themselves, as long as patients get so sick that they cannot attend to their own physical needs, the health-care system will require technically skilled persons to administer medical treatment (especially treatments that must be administered around the clock or to many patients). These situations require devoted and reliable persons to provide constant care for the helpless. So the role of Nurse is not at all obsolete. Of course, it is not clear whether contemporary nurses—the current graduates from our nursing schools—want, or ought to want, to fill that role. However, the role is still there.

If the role of Nurse is coherent, possible, and functional, is it, finally, desirable? Given the obvious drawbacks of the role, so well presented by Dr. Aroskar, should we perhaps conclude that no one ought to fill it? I mentioned above that the traditional functions of the Nurse —administering treatments, providing basic care, and so on—are still essential. But that does not mean that they have to be performed by Nurses. If we decide that the role of Nurse is a sufficiently undesirable one, and that this role should not even be filled by one who desires it, we will simply have to find another way to get those jobs done. There have been roles, after all, in our history, which were abolished even though they easily satisfied the criteria above. The role of "slave," for example, was a highly functional one in our economy until the day it was abandoned; but we were sufficiently convinced that no one, not even one who wanted it very much, should be a slave. It appears that the society was willing to abolish the role and find other ways to get the cotton picked. Is the Nurse a sufficiently dysfunctional role for the individual filling it, and for the practice of health care as a whole, to justify its abolition and replacement with a successor role—say, that of the autonomous professional who is also skilled in nursing practice? Perhaps, as Dr. Aroskar contends, it is that dysfunctional role that damages the autonomy of the individual and deprives the health-care system of the now extensive knowledge of the nursing graduate. But from the point of view of the sick person, there is perhaps an overlooked need for the Nurse. The very flaws and frustrations in the role may turn out to be its major strength in communication with the patient. This line of argument concludes with a brief defense of the Nurse: that, in contrast to the autonomous professional who is suggested as a successor, the Nurse is, or can be, a great comfort to the patient, for she can be sympathetic and supportive while representing no threat to the patient's treatment and autonomy.

Patients are, after all, defined by their suffering. All other individuals in their environment are agents who do things to them, who help them—they are helpless. Their helplessness is measured by their ignorance, over and against the physician's knowledge, and by their abasement, over and against the physician's authority. Patients can do little or nothing to modify their surroundings, within which everything human or mechanical seems to have the right to modify them. The combined weight of this medical mystery and authority is humiliating and oppressive, and patients must often long for relief from them. At the same time, however, except in extraordinary circumstances, patients have no serious question about the worth of what is being done to them, nor any real desire to escape from this expensive oppression. They are fairly sure that, as they have always been taught, it's all for their own good. Patients, then, suffer from a potential conflict between the desire to rebel against treatment and bring it to a halt (to reassert control over their lives), and the desire that treatment should continue (to obtain its benefits). This conflict does not render patients "irrational" in any serious sense, but it may very well render them unhappy, and this peculiar unhappiness, a hospital-produced condition of soul-sickness and discomfort, must be a recurrent feature of the hospital experience. The Nurse, the traditionally subservient handmaiden of the physician, ministers immediately to this condition, by her very definition as well as her skills. If there is a reason to retain her role, this is it. The Nurse is the one who is available for the patients to talk to; the physician has little time to talk. She can listen to complaints indefinitely, sympathize, and even support patients in their rebelliousness; but beyond an occasional timid "Do you want me to tell the Doctor how you feel?" which patients can ignore, the Nurse can do absolutely nothing to modify or terminate their treatment. Since the Nurse has no more control over the environment than patients do, patients can let off steam in perfect safety, knowing that they cannot be taken seriously. Perhaps more importantly, the Nurse's very lack of independence and functional disablement (especially her inability to "follow patients home," i.e., see and treat them outside the hospital) make her a safe recipient for trust and dependence. A patient's privacy is necessarily compromised in any hospital setting, especially with regard to the Nurse. He or she may be unavoidably dependent on the Nurse for personal physical functions which are ordinarily associated with the first and most basic attainment of personal independence, and such dependence is terribly humiliating. The threat to one's autonomy and consequently to one's sense of personal worth is real, and well known. It may be a lot less troublesome when it is personified, not by an autonomous professional who might substitute her decisions for the patient's own, but by a mere Nurse, who just carries out the decisions of others. With no authority of her own, her *de facto* control of patients cannot be a long-term intrusion upon their autonomy. In other words, in a sterile world of authoritative professionals, only the humble, obedient nurse seems to be operating anywhere near the patient's level; she is no threat because she's in the same boat.

The patient, then, may still want and need the Nurse; and I would not be at all surprised to find out that the "public stereotype" of the Nurse is maintained, not just by accident and habit, but by the desire of that public to keep Nurses around for when they get sick. That is, the stereotype may be normative as much as it is empirical. If we find the norm a valid one—if we agree with the public that there should be Nurses—then we should bend our efforts to filling that role with suitable persons. If the current crop of graduate nurses do not want to fill the role, and the indication is that they definitely do not, we are presented with two choices. The first is that graduate nurses will have to fill the role of Nurse, like it or not, for there are no alternatives in present institutions; they should be firmly encouraged to adjust to the role, and the schools they came from should be firmly encouraged to prepare students in the future for careers as Nurses, not as the autonomous professionals fantasized by their frustrated teachers. If that line of approach is repugnant, a second is possible: let them create new roles for themselves, but leave the title of "nurse" for those who will be found to fill the traditional role of the same name. (Perhaps "nurses' aides" would find great satisfaction in assuming the traditional title, duties, and status of the Nurse.) The new roles would be autonomous professional roles, beyond any question, and, as they become available, should fulfill the legitimate aspirations of contemporary nurses for professional careers.

Some move of this sort seems to be taking place now. Dr. Aroskar finds several roles for the new nurse: participant and consultant in the women's health movement, lobbyist, worker for a radically expanded system of free health care, and individual practitioner. In all but the political operations, the nurse in such activities is functioning in an area of care that has only recently been made available to her by expanded training programs for nursing. Right now there may be legis-

ment with Dr. Aroskar that these barriers should fall. New nurses, autonomous professionals regulating their own practices, will occupy these expanded roles; but will they be *nursing* roles? If the designation of "nurse" is dropped from these expanded roles, they can do little to improve nursing's image. On the other hand, they have no problem at all establishing their own images of professional competence and autonomy. The question will have to occur to those dedicated to placing nurses in roles whose image matches their qualifications—is it worth the incalculably long, tedious, and expensive public relations effort to change a deeply entrenched public stereotype that the public may have good reason to want to keep unchanged, when with relative ease the same persons can create new images, not confused with associations of the Nurse, of new occupations in health care, employing their professional skills to meet the expanding needs of the society?

Care of the Sick and Cure of Disease: Comment on "The Fractured Image"

Robert Baker

Professor Aroskar has written an exceptionally rich and insightful essay in which she demonstrates that the prevailing societal view of the nurse is, in the words of the New York State Nurse Practice Act of 1972, that of a "dependent functionary" who, to quote the A.M.A. Committee on Nursing, finds her "logical place at the physician's side" where she acts, "extending the hands of the physician." Dr. Aroskar argues that this conception of the nurse is both sexist and ill informed and seeks further to formulate a sexually neutral model of the nurse's role in which nurses "function independently in the medical sphere."

Her conception of independence is elaborated more fully when she describes the nurse as part of a health-care team in which "each member brings specific as well as overlapping skills to team function."

So what Dr. Aroskar has in mind by the "independence" of the modern nurse is not that of the solo practitioner, but that of a person with a "specific" expertise which can be exercised independently of the expertise of others—that is, of physicians. And, presumably, this expertise might place the nurse in a position of supervising the physician since Dr. Aroskar suggests that membership of the team varies in response to the needs of patient, family, and community and that leadership of the team will also vary according to these needs.

Sceptics, of course, will demand that Dr. Aroskar explain what precisely she has in mind by the "specific" and independent expertise of the nurse. And it is, I think, a weakness in her essay that she does not really suggest wherein that expertise might lie. In what follows I shall try to sketch one way of thinking about nursing which answers the sceptical challenge to Dr. Aroskar's conception of the nurse's role.

Why does the sceptic believe (concurring with the A.M.A. and the State of New York) that the nurse is nothing more than a "dependent functionary"? Dr. Aroskar suggests that sceptics hold this view because they are sexist. Most physicians are male, 98 percent of all nurses, female. Hence, the nurse role is naturally conceptualized as a feminine, dependent role—an auxiliary to the dominant male role of the physician.

The problem with this analysis of those sceptical of a new, independent role for nursing is that, even if the analysis is entirely accurate, it is irrelevant to the logical force of the sceptic's argument. For while it is undeniably true that, traditionally, nursing has been regarded as a feminine role, it is not at all clear whether the role of nurse is seen as dependent because it is filled by females, who are held to be incapable of independent action by a male-dominated, sexist society (as Dr. Aroskar would, no doubt, contend), *or* whether females have been channeled into nursing because the profession, *by its very nature*, requires its members to play a dependent and subservient role (i.e., the traditional female role in a sexist society). Hence the facts that almost all nurses are female, that the traditional nurse's role is feminine, and that our society has traditionally been sexist, neither support nor undercut scepticism about the new role of nursing.

The only proper way to reply to the sceptic's challenge is to demonstrate how a nurse could have "specific" expertise that might make her the equal of or the occasional superior to physicians, or both. In order to do this it is helpful to ask, "Why does the sceptic believe that it is impossible for the nurse to act as anything but a dependent extension of the physician's hand?" The likely answer is to be found in the popular conception of sickness and health care. It is generally held that to be sick is to have a disease (such as influenza, diabetes, or cancer) and that one goes to a health-care worker, typically a doctor, to be cured of this disease. The doctor has studied science, diseases, and medicine at college, medical school, during internship and residency—in fact, for at least a decade since high school. The nurse need only have studied for two years after high school—and she seems to have studied essentially the same subjects as the physician. How then can the nurse hope to be anything but a dependent extension of the physician's hands? How could she possibly be an equal partner with the physician as part of a health-care team, much less his occasional superior? Wherein could her special expertise possibly lie?

The sociologist Talcott Parsons was one of the first to suggest that this popular conception of medicine is altogether too simple. He thought that one must make a distinction between *sickness*, on the one hand, and *biophysiological occurrences* on the other. Following in Parsons' footsteps, I should like to distinguish between *disease* and *sickness*. "Disease" is a scientific, causal term which refers to a condition where some part, element, or subsystem of an organism goes awry so that it has caused or will cause the organism to enter a state which contravenes that organism's own interests. Traditionally the cause is thought of as pathology, the effects as symptoms. And, in the traditional view, the function of a doctor is either to restore the pathological condition to normal, or, failing that, to alleviate the symptoms caused by the pathology. Thus, insofar as medicine is concerned only with the curing of pathological conditions and/or the amelioration of symptoms, it can be nothing more than a practical extension of physiology and biochemistry.

"Sickness," however, is another concept. It is quite possible to be diseased but not sick, but it is not possible (as I use these terms) to be sick but not diseased. By "sickness" I mean a task or role incapacity caused and maintained by a disease; thus *someone is held to be sick if having a disease makes the person incapable of performing the tasks or roles (which one expects that person to perform)*. If a would-be Romeo finds his acne preventing him from playing the lover, he has a dermatological sickness. But a man with diabetes who takes insulin for his disease, and can then do anything he wants, is not sick (even if he has exactly the same acne condition as the would-be Romeo).

Sickness is a relative concept. Conditions that make a weightlifter sick (e.g., a sprained wrist) might not phase a college lecturer, and, conversely, the laryngitis that would incapacitate a lecturer might not even inconvenience the weightlifter. Sickness is not, however, a subjective phenomenon; for it is an objective fact that sprain makes the weightlifter incapable of lifting weights, just as laryngitis prevents the lecturer from lecturing. Nor is sickness a matter of physiology or of biochemistry, for tasks and roles are neither physiological nor biochemical in nature. While disease may be a matter of biochemistry and physiology, sickness cannot be. Therefore it follows that insofar as the task of medicine is to heal the sick, it is not and cannot be merely a matter of biochemistry. Hence since medicine deals with sickness as well as disease, not all medical expertise is strictly scientific.

Who has a greater knowledge of the tasks and roles that shape a patient's life, the hospital physician or the hospital nurse? Who has more contact with the patient and the family, the specialist, or the nursing staff? In many cases the answer will be the patient's doctor (especially if the doctor is a family practitioner who has taken care of the patient for many years) but, typically, those who have the greatest contact, who best know the patient's ambitions, desires, tasks, and roles, hence, his or her sickness, are the nurses. Thus, by the very nature of his or her job the nurse tends to have more special expertise about the patient's *sickness* than the physician. Hence, wherever such knowledge is significant for patient care, the nursing staff should have an independent input into the decisions of a health-care team; and where considerations of sickness override those of disease, the nursing staff should have the predominant role in the decisions of the health-care team.

It might be asked, how could considerations of sickness ever override those of disease? Actually such considerations are frequently crucial, for it should always be remembered that disease is significant only because it makes people sick. I shall, however, consider one clear case in which sickness is more significant than disease, one case in which the expertise of the nurse is more important than that of the physician—the case of the incurable, hospitalized patient.

When a patient is recognized as incurable, as "beyond help," he or she is not beyond the help of nurses, only of physicians, for by their declaration of incurability physicians have admitted that nothing can be done to ameliorate sickness. But if death is inevitable, pain and incapacity need not be, and the tasks and roles that they set for themselves help incurable patients satisfy their own, often internal, task-role expectations as much as they possibly can. The role of the nurse is to care for the sick in their sickness, even when cure is impossible.

The description of the role of the nurse in health-care teams that care for the incurably ill may seem unduly abstract or outrageously idealistic to some. Yet it is a reasonably accurate description of St. Christopher's and other hospices. St. Christopher's is a nursing facility for the incurably ill directed by Cicely Saunders—a nurse who, in order to have her theories of nursing the incurably ill listened to, had to qualify as a physician. At St. Christopher's, care of the sick is primary; disease *per se* is untreated, and physicians are indeed ancillary to nurses.

There are, then, both in theory and in practice places where the nurse's role as care provider for the sick is properly predominant over the physician's role as a disease expert. More often, disease is as important as, sometimes even more important than, sickness—and hence it is proper for doctors to be as important as, sometimes even more important than, nurses. The relative importance of the roles is less significant, in the context of this chapter, than the demonstration of the fact that Professor Aroskar is undoubtedly correct in arguing that the nurse can and should be something more than an "extension of the physician's hands." The nurse can be, and ought to be, an expert at caring for the sick, which makes nurses separate from, and sometimes more than equal to, physicians, and certainly, therefore, superior to the physician's hands.

NOTES

1. Simmons, Leo W., "Past and Potential Images of the Nurse," *Nursing Forum*, 1:19, Summer 1962.

2. *Ibid.*, pp. 21-22.

3. Olesen, Virginia L. and Whittaker, Elvi W., *The Silent Dialogue: A Study in the Social Psychology of Professional Socialization*, San Francisco: Jossey-Bass, Inc., 1968, pp. 126-27.

4. Simmons, *Image of the Nurse*, pp. 24-30.

5. Beletz, Elaine E., "The Public Image: A Devoted Heart, Disciplined Hand, Not Necessarily An Inquiring Mind!" *Imprint*, 2:41, April 1976.

6. _____. "Is Nursing's Public Image Up to Date?" *Nursing Outlook*, 22:434, July 1974.

7. *Ibid.*, p. 435.

8. Vaz, Dolores, "High School Senior Boys' Attitudes Toward Nursing as a Career," *Nursing Research*, 17:533-38, November-December 1968.

9. Mauksch, Hans O., "Nursing: Churning for Change," in Freeman, Howard E., et al. (eds.) *Handbook of Medical Sociology*, 2nd ed., Englewood Cliffs, N.J.: Prentice-Hall, Inc., 1972, p. 208.

10. Hudspeth, Randy, "Will the Real Nurse Please Stand Up?" *Imprint*, 2:22, April 1976.

11. Wheelock, Alan, "The Tarnished Image," *Nursing Outlook*, 24:509-10, August 1976.

12. Mauksch, *Nursing: Churning for Change*, p. 223.

13. Woodham-Smith, Cecil, *Lonely Crusader: The Life of Florence Nightingale*, New York: Bantam Books, 1963, p. 32.

14. *Ibid.*, p. 35.

15. *Ibid.*, p. 62.

16. *Ibid.*, pp. 166-67.

17. *Ibid.*, p. 172.

18. *Ibid.*, p. 73.

19. Ashley, Jo Ann, *Hospitals, Paternalism, and the Role of the Nurse*, New York: Teachers College Press, 1976, p. 5.

20. *Ibid.*, p. 9.

21. *Ibid.*, p. 35.

22. *Ibid.*, p. 11.

23. *Ibid.*, p. 35.

24. *Ibid.*, pp. 106-7.

25. *Ibid.*, p. 107.

26. *Ibid.*, p. 17.

27. Duff, Raymond S. and Hollingshead, August B., *Sickness and Society*, New York: Harper and Row, Publishers, 1968, p. 78.

28. *Ibid.*, pp. 373-74.

29. Jacox, Ada, "Professional Socialization of Nurses," *Journal of the New York State Nurses Association*, 4:8, November 1973.

30. Simmons, *Image of the Nurse*, pp. 25-26.

31. Fox, David J., Diamond, Lorraine K. and Associates, *Satisfying and Stressful Situations in Basic Programs in Nursing Education*, New York: Bureau of Publications, Teachers College, Columbia University, 1964, pp. 198-207.

32. Davis, Anne J., "Self-Concept, Occupational Role Expectations, and Occupational Choice in Nursing and Social Work," *Nursing Research*, 18:57, January-February 1969.

33. DeLora, Jack R. and Moses, Dorothy V., "Specialty Preferences and Characteristics of Nursing Students in Baccalaureate Programs," *Nursing Research*, 18:137, March-April 1969.

34. Kramer, Marlene. *Reality Shock: Why Nurses Leave Nursing*. Saint Louis: C. V. Mosby Co., 1974.

35. Murphy, Catherine P. *Levels of Moral Reasoning in a Selected Group of Nursing Practitioners*. Unpublished doctoral dissertation, Teachers College, Columbia University, 1976.

36. Ashley, *Role of the Nurse*, pp. 116-17.

37. Hall, Virginia C., "The Legal Scope of Nurse Practitioners under Nurse Practice and Medical Practice Acts," in Bliss, Ann S. and Cohen, Eva D. (eds.), *The New Health Professionals*. Germantown, Md.: Aspen Systems Corporation, 1977, pp. 110-11.

38. *Ibid.*, p. 112.

39. O'Dell, Margaret L., "Physicians' Perceptions of an Extended Role for the Nurse," *Nursing Research*, 23:348:51, July-August 1974.

40. Chesler, Phyllis, *Women and Madness*, Garden City, N.Y.: Doubleday & Company, 1972, pp. 67-68.

41. *Ibid.*, pp. 68-69.

42. Stein, Leonard I., "The Doctor-Nurse Game," in Lewis, Edith R. (ed.), *Changing Patterns of Nursing Practice: New Needs, New Roles*, New York: The American Journal of Nursing Company, 1971, p. 227.

43. *Ibid.*, pp. 228-29.

44. *Ibid.*, pp. 233-34.

45. Dickoff, James and James, Patricia, "Beliefs and Values: Bases for Curriculum Design," *Nursing Research*, 19:425, September, October 1970.

46. Chioni, Rose M. and Panicucci, Carol, "Tomorrow's Nurse Practitioners," in Lewis, Edith R., (ed.), *Changing Patterns of Nursing Practice: New Needs, New Roles*, New York: The American Journal of Nursing Company, 1971, pp. 106-107.

47, Brown, Esther L. *Nursing Reconsidered: A Study of Change*, Part 2. Philadelphia: J. B. Lippincott Company, 1971.

48. Simmons, *Image of the Nurse*, pp. 17-18.

49. Gardner, Harold. "Joint Practice: A New Dimension in Nurse Physician Collaboration," *American Journal of Nursing*, 77:1466-68, September 1977.

BIBLIOGRAPHY

Baker, R. "Mental Illness Defined" in *Encyclopedia of Bioethics*, New York: Free Press, 1978.

Baker, R. and Elliston, F. *Philosophy and Sex*, Buffalo: Prometheus Books, 1976.

Parsons, T. "Definitions of Health and Illness in the Light of American Values and Social Structure" in E. Gautley Jaco (ed.), *Patients, Physicians, and Illness*, New York: The Free Press, 1958.

Saunders, C. "Care for the Dying," *Patient Care*, Vol. 3, No. 6, June 1976, *The Management of Terminal Illness*, Hospital Publications Ltd., London, 1967.

[3]

Value-Laden Technologies and the Politics of Nursing

Sandra Harding

Does the contemporary technology of medicine increase or decrease the quality of the health care we receive? What might nurses do to increase the benefits of the modern technologies of medicine? Is "caring," or even "curing," really a necessary or a legitimate goal for nurses, given the modern technology of health care?

These are the obvious questions to ask about how modern technology affects nursing. These questions reflect our perceptions that visits to hospitals and even to doctors' offices are frequently more depressing than they need be. They also reflect our suspicions that perhaps we have the wrong set of expectations about modern nursing. Perhaps caring and curing are now historically inappropriate goals for nurses to have. The curing seems to be almost entirely the job of the doctor, his drugs, and his machines. The caring seems to be something that modern, scientific health care shouldn't be expected to provide.

However, I do not think these questions or the suspicions they reflect can be usefully addressed until we have a critical understanding both of the nature of technological decisions and of the structure of contemporary nursing. The first part of this chapter will examine what is wrong with three traditional ways of understanding technology. In the second part, a more adequate conception of technology will be used to illuminate the effect of technological decisions on medical practice today, and, especially, on nursing. At the end of the chapter I shall return to suggest the different set of questions we need to ask about how nurses might respond to the technological choices which have structured contemporary health care.

THE NATURE OF TECHNOLOGY

Traditionally, technology has been understood with respect to its social value. Technology is thought of either as autonomous—as providing its own ends—or as a value-neutral means to ends which are chosen entirely in the moral/political arena. Those who think of technology as autonomous divide into utopians and dystopians. Only if we see what is wrong with these three simplistic and false views of technology can we formulate a conception of technology adequate to enable us to answer our questions about the technology of health care.

Utopians claim that technological change intrinsically leads to a decrease in pain, suffering, exploitation, and oppression, and to an expansion of human opportunities and of our powers over our own fate. Such utopian views are both ancient and modern—they were dominant most recently in the 1960s. In 1968, C. West Churchman said, "We have the technological capacity of adequately feeding, sheltering, and clothing every inhabitant of the world." We can provide "adequate medical care" and "sufficient education" for everyone. He continues, "we have the technological capability of outlawing warfare," of maximizing "freedom of opinion and freedom of action," and of "organizing the societies of the world" to discern and carry out these solutions.[1] In his illuminating study of attitudes toward technology, Bernard Gendron points out how in various ways, Churchman's optimism was echoed in the 1960s by John Kenneth Galbraith, Robert McNamara, Walt Rostow, Buckminster Fuller, John Maynard Keynes, Arthur Clarke, C.P. Snow, Alvin Toffler, Herman Kahn, and B.F. Skinner.[2]

In contrast, dystopians see technology as an intrinsically regressive social force. Technology dehumanizes us, alienates us from ourselves, from each other, and from nature. It curtails our choices and subverts our freedoms. Gendron distinguishes the classical and the counterculture dystopians. Classical dystopians such as Dostoevski, Huxley, and Orwell saw technology as bringing in its wake oppressive political repercussions. The "Brave New World" of the future would be a "nightmare of total organization," as Huxley described it. Jacques Ellul, Herbert Marcuse, and Robert Heilbroner have also shared in this view. The more recent "counterculture dystopians" such as Theodore Roszak, Philip Slater, and Charles Reich argue that it is the imperatives of modern technology that are responsible for the growth of psychological alienation in contemporary life.[3]

Let me stress that both utopians and dystopians assume that technological change is an autonomous, independently existing force which determines its own ends.[4] This conception of technological change encourages the view that all humans can do is increase or decrease the amount of technological change in a society. For utopians, the more the better. For dystopians, we must hold back the wheels of so-called progress and return to a simpler life, closer to nature, where each individual's life had greater meaning and dignity.

In opposition to the utopian and dystopian conceptions of technology as intrinsically value-laden are those who see technology merely as a means. Technological choices are value-neutral. It is only the ends to which a technology is put which are value-laden. From this perspective, it is thought that one and the same technology can be used for good or ill. Thus no one need worry about the characteristics of a technology itself, but only about the moral and political goals of those who make use of a particular technological alternative.

Each of these three views of the nature of technology denies that the other two are correct, so at most one of them could be true. But I think that none of these views is correct. I shall not present lengthy arguments against the utopian and dystopian views on the assumption that their oversimplifications are obvious. It should be clear that technological change has both good and bad aspects—it is neither automatically liberating nor automatically oppressive. And, it is clear that moral and political choices in the community do influence in part whether a technological alternative will be used well or ill, so the shared assumption that technology is an autonomous force is not justified.

The third conception of technology is also inadequate. Technology is not value-neutral. This third conception depends upon two questionable though widespread assumptions. The first is that technology is merely an adjunct or product of science. Thus value-neutralists usually mean by "technology" not a force but a thing—tools, machines, instruments, appliances, "hardware." In Langdon Winner's terms, they mean an "apparatus."[5] For instance, one author writes of "the instruments and machines used by the contemporary physician" which constitute a "therapeutic technology."[6] But it becomes clear that he means instruments and machines used also by other health workers under the direction of the physician. Thus the "therapeutic technology" includes the machines *and* their operators, nurses, technicians, and others. Another example of this tendency can be found in an essay entitled "Evaluating the Physician and His Technology," where "his technology" is stated to include hardware such as "computerized X-ray scanners" and "fiberoptic endoscopes," but, of course it turns out that it also includes the workers who operate the hardware.[7] When technology is thought of simply as one of the "products" of scientific research, it is easy to assume that it consists only of machines and instruments which are themselves value-neutral. But technological alternatives involve not only choices between machines and instruments, but also between techniques and skilled procedures, and also between ways to organize the people using the instruments in particular techniques. If one wishes to avoid confronting value questions, it is comforting and useful to think of technology merely as value-free hardware.

The second questionable assumption is that a significant feature of the science producing technology is its value-neutrality. Science is "pure"; it is only when the results of science are socially applied in one way or another that there are positive or negative social consequences. Thus the scientist—and, by association, the technician—need not be concerned with social values. Social values are a matter of morality and politics, and both of these are realms where the special talents of the scientist and technician are not relevant to making choices. The scientist or technician *qua* scientist or technician can provide information, but not make moral or political choices. Science and technology are matters of research, theory, and the mechanical construction of instruments and machines. The two worlds are entirely separate, and the concerns of one realm should not be allowed to intrude perniciously upon the other. Technological choices share in the ability of science to be value-neutral. This view of science as value-neutral has been widely criticized. I think it is a false view, though I cannot argue that here.[8] So these two questionable assumptions—that "technology" means some sort of hardware, and that the science producing this "hardware" is itself value-neutral—support the view that technology is value-neutral. These assumptions prevent us from understanding the much more complex and interesting relationship between technological decisions and moral/political decisions.

A more adequate conception of technology emerges when we think of technologies as ways of organizing human labor which are influenced both by the sophistication of the apparatuses and technology available, and also by the moral and political goals dominant in a society. Technological decisions are in part moral/political decisions (vs. the utopians and dystopians), though only some technological alternatives are compatible with any given moral/political goal (vs. the value-neutralists). The two-way interaction between the development of apparatuses and techniques and the prevailing moral/political values is thus much more active than the traditional conceptions of technology lead us to believe. New technologies and new moral/political values often emerge together. To the extent that we understand this, we have it in our power consciously to choose technologies which will advance desirable moral/political values. Ignorance condemns us to live out the consequences of others' choices.

Any kind of labor may be organized in a variety of ways with or without tools or hardware. Tilling the soil may be done by large numbers of slaves who use short-handle hoes and work on plantations, by housewives using long hoes in home gardens, by tenant farmers using mule-drawn plows, by owners of small farms using tractor-drawn plows, or by paid laborers operating huge combines for an agricultural conglomerate. All of these are technologies of farming. Which one we should expect to find at a given time and place is a matter in part of the sophistication of the tools and techniques available to a culture. It is also a matter of what kinds of political relations are desired by those in a position to make their choices felt. And, to complicate the matter, the sophistication of the tools and of the techniques available to a culture is in part a matter of the prevailing political values. So political values influence the development of, as well as the choice between, technological alternatives and technological choices influence the political values in a society. Let me give an example of each kind of case and then an illustration of the complexity of the interaction between technological choices and political values.

Tilling the soil with a short-handle hoe is inherently dehumanizing. It requires backbreaking physical labor to produce the food necessary for maintaining life. But in spite of this obviously brutal character of hand-hoe farming, many societies would have little motivation to develop more mechanically sophisticated forms of agriculture. Their hierarchical political structures can be maintained only if certain technologies remain relatively primitive. Over 35 years ago, Edgar Zilsel pointed out some of the social conditions necessary for the development of "machinery and science":

> Machinery and science cannot develop in a civilization based on slave labor. Slaves generally are unskilled and cannot be entrusted with handling complex devices. Moreover, slave labor seems to be cheap enough to make introduction of machines superfluous. On the other hand, slavery makes the social contempt for manual work so strong that it cannot be overcome by the educated.[9]

Zilsel does not say that the lack of slave labor is *sufficient* for the development of machinery and science—only that it is *necessary*. Thus political values influence the development of technological alternatives.

But the causal influences go in the other direction as well. Liberating technologies are conducive to more democratic political structures. For instance, it is difficult to underestimate the long-run and short-run political consequences of the invention and widespread distribution of cheap, efficient contraceptives. It is clear that this technology of birth-control has the effect of eliminating for women the heretofore virtually inevitable connection between women's expression of their sexuality and pregnancy. No longer are women doomed to the endless labor of pregnancies and child-raising as a "career," a labor which has been easily manipulated socially to keep women as second-class citizens—discriminated against in education, occupational choices, and political expression. When women are free from endless pregnancies and childcare it is harder to manipulate them into remaining second-class citizens. As is plainly visible in American culture, changes in political values in matters affecting women are underway, and the new technology of contraception has influenced the direction of change. Technological choices influence political values.

The complexity of the interaction between technological choice and political values can be seen if we look at yet another case in which an available and potentially liberating technology was perverted to oppressive uses. Recently several historians of technology have been examining two reconceptualizations of housework in the present century which succeeded in keeping women at home in tedious domestic drudgery just when housework could have been organized so as to release women from this demeaning work so that they could enter the paid labor force. In "The Manufacture of Housework," Barbara Ehrenreich and Deirdre English examine the emergence of the "domestic science" movement around the turn of the century. In "Two Washes in the Morning and a Bridge Party at Night: The American Housewife Between the Wars," Ruth Schwartz Cowan studies the emergence of the "domestic art" movement in the 1920s.[10] In their essays, these historians are concerned with the puzzling fact that while the development and mass marketing of labor-saving devices in the late 19th and early 20th centuries should have reduced the amount of labor required to maintain the household, "women's work" did not significantly decrease during this period. In fact, in at least one area of domestic work, laundering, the time devoted to it has actually increased over the past half-century—and this is the period which saw the introduction of the washer, the dryer, and wash-and-wear clothing. In fact, decisions about how to organize domestic labor—decisions about which domestic technology to promote—were made in accordance with the so-called public interest. As Ehrenreich, English, and Cowan point out, these interests were not defined by women themselves. They were defined by the owners of industries who needed the emerging class system stabilized so that hungry and relatively docile workers would be appropriately socialized and tended, by the producers of household equipment who needed ever-increasing markets for their goods, and by other needs of the "public institutions" of 20th-century American life. These are the institutions from which women's voices have been barred. In this case, the technology was already developed which could have liberated women from domestic labor, but political values insured that this technological potential would be perverted to maintain a class of workers with little political power. It has taken almost a century for women to figure out that fighting dirt in a color-coordinated kitchen isn't going to bring much happiness in life, that this is not an adequate substitute for performing meaningful work in the public world.

We do not live in a slave society. But we do live in a society where many people have little chance to participate in the decision-making which crucially affects the quality of their lives. Political change is a prerequisite for using well the technological alternatives available to us. Thus I am arguing that technological changes contribute to human freedom only when they further projects selected by the workers themselves (and we are all workers). Social conflict will be the necessary result of trying to force technological changes to bring about goals detrimental to workers' interests. Thus a political system that encourages technological changes benefiting special interests which are inconsistent with general social needs is, to that extent, an illegitimate political system. In our society, in many cases, special interests have been supported through a privileged, technocratic leadership. These leaders monopolize technical knowledge and thus "automatically" become a class of decision-makers who make decisions for everyone, even when their interests are in conflict with the interests of the majority.[11] Inadequate conceptualizations of technology both contribute to ineffective and destructive interactions with nature and also support privileged access to the social benefits of technological change. I have argued that we should conceive of a technology as a way of organizing human labor which is influenced both by the sophistication of the apparatuses and techniques available, and also influenced by the moral and political goals of the society. With this in mind, we may now ask how the labor of contemporary health care is organized in our society. Whose interests have directed the vast changes visible recently? How has nursing been shaped by these changes? How might nurses influence the direction of technological change in health care?

THE ORGANIZATION OF HEALTH CARE

Health care has been organized in a variety of ways, as the history and sociology of medicine reveal. In our society health care is organized around hospitals and vast numbers of hierarchically-organized workers—from research physicians to nurses' aides. Nurses themselves exist at several intermediate levels in this hierarchy. In the following account, the outlines of which are no doubt familiar to many readers, I wish to bring out some peculiar and significant features of nursing which are easy to overlook if one fails to see the function nursing performs within the overall structure of health care. The organization of the labor of nursing is grasped, I shall argue, only if one understands nursing as an industrialized form of traditional women's work. Thus the position of nursing is located in the structure of health care in much the same way as domestic labor is situated in the structure of social life in general. In particular, the service ethic which in part attracts women to nursing is "cooled out" for lower levels of nurses through techniques of industrial management and in part through the substitution of a "professional" ethic for the service ethic. These subversions of the service ethic result in nurses' "natural" social strengths as well as their training being turned against them and against those they are charged to care for and cure. I turn first to remind you of the particular way the labor of nursing has been organized.

Educated women employed outside the home have tended to cluster in the so-called helping professions. In addition to nursing, the most obvious of these occupations are secretarial work, teaching, social work, psychology, and the paramedical services of occupational, physical, and speech therapy. There are two reasons for this clustering. First of all, women have had few other options for paid employment. Secondly, all of these jobs call upon the social strengths women have developed in their traditional roles in the family—nurturing, caring, doing the "housekeeping" tasks. In the helping professions the social strengths of women are mobilized on behalf not just of the family but of the whole society.[12] The negative side of this segregation of the work force is that until very recently women have been systematically prevented from entering not only any areas of the work force where they might obtain high salaries, but also any areas where their duties would not be consistent with their feminine roles in the family.

They have been especially prevented from entering any of the policy-making roles in the economy, in government, in education, and in health care.

It is no accident that the helping professions emerged on a significant scale in the middle of the 19th century. They can be seen as the psychosocial counterpart of the move in material production which relocated economic activity out of the small-scale and personal atmosphere of the individual home and into the large-scale and impersonal setting of the factory. The trend in both material production and in the production of services has been toward breaking down complex production processes into increasingly· specialized and repetitive activities. This division of labor and accompanying specialization is necessary if there is to be centralized control of production processes. And centralized control is necessary if just a few people are to extract the maximum profit from the labor of production which is performed mainly by others. The particular recent forms of industrialization of the production of both material goods and psychosocial services have been useful for the accumulation of both political power and wealth by a minority of people. In the case of health care, the hospital has become the hub of the wheel of the production of services, and it is here that the structure and value of nursing are most obvious.

There are two striking features that nursing shares with the other kinds of women's work, including the domestic labor from which it emerged. The first of these is the contradiction between the social value of the work and the public recognition of this value. The second is the way that the service ethic—the ethic of altruism that is in part responsible for attracting women to nursing—is "cooled out" and subverted. It is "cooled out" in different ways for different ranks of nurses. As long as they are not recognized, these "cooling out" devices prevent nurses from organizing to change the conditions of their labor—that is, from organizing to change the technologies under which health-care is delivered. Thus nursing is like other kinds of women's work in that the special strengths of women are turned against both women themselves and against those for whom they are expected to care.

I turn first to the contradiction between the social value of nursing and the public recognition of this value. This contradiction appears once we note the three features which distinguish the labor of health care from other kinds of industrial labor. First of all, the introduction of a new technology—a new way of organizing labor—makes most industries less labor-intensive. Such "substitute technologies" allow the production of more goods with less human labor. However, technological change in health care has required the hiring and training of vast numbers of additional workers to operate the various new machines and instruments. At the same time, the full number of existing staff is required to provide the continuing services. This increase in the health-care work force is due to the "add-on" character of most of the technological changes in health care. These changes do not merely substitute a new way of accomplishing a task for an old way but, instead, accomplish things not possible before.[13] The number of workers needed to provide health care has vastly increased, and the greatest increase has been in the lower-level workers—nurses, technicians, and nurses' aides.

Secondly, the social value of health care is immediately and unquestionably obvious.[14] It is obvious first to the workers themselves. The factory worker may wonder about the value of a new flavor of cat food or about the value of the 19th brand of can opener she is involved in producing, but health is a "product" the value of which is immediately apparent to health-care workers. The social value of health care is also perfectly clear to everyone else in the society: we wonder about the value of the cat food or the can opener, but we never question the value of health. We want it, and the more of it the better. And who provides all of this valuable health care? While only 8 percent of health-care workers are doctors, 50 percent are nurses. The remaining 42 percent is divided among the fields of dentistry, pharmacy, clinical laboratory services, environmental control, secretarial and office services, and various other miscellaneous categories.[15] This, too, is obvious to the nurses themselves, if less so to the rest of society. A nurse in a municipal hospital says with only slight exaggeration: "You could imagine a hospital with no doctors. Everything would get done just the same. But try to imagine a hospital with no nurses. It would be chaos. The patients would all die of neglect."[16]

In the third place, in the "factory" of health care, the hospital, there is extraordinary functional interdependence among workers who have very different rank within the hospital and very different social status in the outside world. This too distinguishes health-care workers from other industrial workers.

> A surgical operation commonly requires the cooperative efforts of a team whose members range in rank from surgeon to aides. The surgeon has had eight or more years of post-college training; he may earn more than $50,000 a year and sit on one of the hospital's key management committees, on the almost all-powerful medical board or even on the board of directors. The aides may have no high school education, earn less than $7000, and lack even the authority to make a simple suggestion. But in the operation itself they are both essential participants, as the aide can easily demonstrate by making a small but fatal mistake.[17]

The nurse's contribution to health care is as crucial as that of any other health-care worker. This contradiction in the nurse's importance and her rank in the hospital hierarchy is mirrored by the contradiction in the doctor's importance and his rank in the hospital hierarchy. Given his *functional* importance, the doctor has a vastly inflated status within the hospital. As the technology of health care becomes increasingly that of an industrial assembly line, the doctor more and more becomes just one among many production workers, one skilled worker among many. He works right alongside the nurses, aides, and technicians and his work is continually observed by these, his inferiors in rank. It is these "inferiors," and usually they alone, who are witnesses to all of his failures—his faulty diagnoses, unnecessary postoperative complications, and the like.[18] But, as an integral part of hospital management, he has the highest rank in the institution.

Nurses are low paid and many of the mundane jobs doctors used to do have been transferred to nurses. The division of labor in health care is spectacular. And narrow job definitions are enforced through hierarchical control within the health system. A nurse writes in the journal *Nursing Outlook*:

> So often I knew the patient better than the physician and had scientifically based reasons for wanting to initiate a certain action—yet I was prevented from doing so without being given equally valid reasons. The goal seemed to be to keep the institution operating at a smooth pace and to placate the other professional people, rather than to help the patient to meet his needs.[19]

Individual nurses perform an increasingly small portion of the process of producing health care. As with any labor industrialized in this way, it becomes easy for workers to lose sight of the final "product" of such specialized labor. Nurses report again and again the vast gap between what they are capable of and trained to do on the one hand, and what in fact the hierarchy of hospital work allows them to do on the other hand. One nurse says: "We're really like secretaries pushing papers around. All we do is dispense pills to the patients."[20] And a nurse educator with 12 years nursing experience behind her says:

> Let's face it, nursing is a rotten job. You have no control over hours, you rotate shifts, work weekends and holidays. You get moved from floor to floor. Sometimes you're the only one with fifty patients and yet the supervisor comes in and yells at you and you think, what do they expect from me?[21]

In this respect, nursing is organized exactly like the rest of "women's work." Thus the high social value of the huge contribution of nurses to health care is not rewarded in commensurable income, appropriate social status inside or outside the institution, or proportionate control over either the working conditions of nursing or the way in general in which health care is delivered.

The second striking feature nursing shares with other kinds of women's work is the way that the social ethic is "cooled out" and subverted. It is cooled out in different ways for different ranks of nurses, ways appropriate to their social statuses in the larger society—their "absolute" social statuses.

This preservation of absolute social status in the ranked divison of labor inside the hospital is characteristic of hospital workers in general. Doctors are 98 percent white, 93 percent male, and predominantly from upper and upper-middle class families. Nurses and technicians are usually lower-middle class and white; 98 percent of nurses and about 70 percent of technicians are women. Aides, cooks, and maids are the lower-class men and women. In the big northern cities these are usually black, Chicano, or Puerto Rican. In New York City's municipal hospitals, for instance, between 80 and 90 percent are nonwhite.[22] The preservation of different absolute statuses within the nursing ranks insures that nurses will find it difficult to identify and to organize around shared goals.

For the practical nurses, nurses' aides, and other health-care workers in the lower ranks of the hospital hierarchy, the hierarchical control of the conditions under which health care is delivered eventually alienates them from the content of their work. As the Ehrenreichs report:

> Conditions (in even the best hospitals), however, are enough to undermine the efforts of even the most dedicated workers—understaffing, inadequate supplies and equipment, obstructive red tape, priorities given to non-patient care functions, etc. In their training or orientation, lower-level workers are warned against taking it all too seriously. "Do not try to achieve perfection in everything, because, admirable as it is, it is an invitation to failure and often is most impracticable," warns one text for practical nurses. (*Personal and Vocational Relationships in Practical Nursing*, Carmen F. Ross, Philadelphia 1969, p. 103.) Suggestions and innovations from the ranks are not encouraged, and are usually viewed as "troublemaking." An aide told us, "You go to your supervisor [about a patient care problem]. She doesn't do anything. Eventually, *you* stop caring, too." Again and again we heard the refrain. "After a while you just don't give a damn." You become the adjusted, "industrialized" worker for whom hospital work is just a job.[23]

Through techniques of "industrial management," workers at the lower levels of nursing are forced to accept and adjust to the class divisions preserved within health care, and to deny the service ethic which was in part responsible for attracting them to health care.

One might think that the recent trend toward unionization of hospital workers would alleviate this situation. However, unions do not challenge either the way work is organized or the nature or quality of the "product" workers produce. As in other unions, hospital unions succeed—when they do—simply in getting more pay for jobs no matter how meaningless and dead-end they are. And as in other industries, hospitals pass on to consumers the wage increases won by unions. Thus by failing to challenge the organization of health-care labor or the nature of the health care "produced," unions in fact force the needs of the worker to be in conflict with the needs of the consumer of health care.[24] This can be regarded as the final subversion of the service ethic.

On the other hand, for higher-level health workers such as registered nurses, the ideology of professionalism leads them to deny the class divisions among health-care workers and to divert their service ethic into a professional "ethic."[25] In the professional "ethic" it is not service to the patient—caring and curing—but loyalty to the institution which guides their perception of and ability to deliver health care.

This is not a description of the professional "ethic" that is likely to comfort professionals, because the ideal to which professionals overtly pay allegiance is a very different one. Just a few years ago, as astute a social observer as Paul Goodman though it uncontroversial to say that "professionals are autonomous individuals beholden to the nature of things and the judgment of their peers, and bound by an explicit or implicit oath to benefit their clients and the community."[26] This ideal has been a powerful social force motivating many who have entered law, medicine, and university life. Has the ideal really functioned to guide professionals in serving the needs of clients and community? A skeptical answer to this question has been emerging from recent examinations of the struggles of the rising middle class in 19th-century America.

The first clue toward understanding how professions in fact function is to note that from a legal point of view a profession is a monopoly: ". . . a profession is an organized occupational group which has been granted a monopoly over the performance of certain functions and a certain degree of autonomy in carrying them out."[27] Among the monopolies the medical profession has been granted are exclusive rights to police medical workers, to set standards for entering the various fields of medical work, to practice surgery, to prescribe drugs, to classify people as fit or unfit for various duties or functions.[28] From a historical perspective, these monopolies on professional services emerged as the middle class sought to entrench its interests institutionally. In one of the recent studies, Burton Bledstein argues that the "cult of professionalism" emerged only with the help of the developing modern university, catering to middle-class students and finding it profitable to promote its role as gatekeeper to the profession. The modern university provides the foundation for the "true professionals" who insist that equality of opportunity and that democratic goals are identical with meritocratic ones. Since "merit will always find its true reward," professionals can confidently identify life with work and career. Since their high social status is taken as a reflection of that invisible hand of fate correctly rewarding merit, they can pride themselves on the way in which they bring both native talent and subsequent training to solve crucial social problems, simultaneously advancing both themselves and the interests of society at large.[29]

When we consider nursing, it becomes apparent that nurses have never even been encouraged to be professionals in Goodman's ideal sense at all. Bound by the rules of institutional hierarchy, they are allowed neither to function as autonomous individuals "beholden to the nature of things," nor, consequently, to act in accordance with what they perceive to be the greatest benefit for their patients and the community. Moreover, in the legal sense, nursing has only the most superficial resemblance to its presumably by definition coequal sibling professions. Like members of all the other "health professions" except for doctors, registered nurses as a group are in fact subordinate to and supervised by the medical profession itself.[30] The ideology of RNs requires that they recognize their "proper place" in the hierarchy of health care.

While the 19th-century emergence of the modern university and of the professions strengthened the ability of doctors to control the organization of health care, the "battle between the sexes" in medicine had been lost by women long before that time. Women were told their "proper place" in medicine repeatedly throughout the last four centuries. Women physicians and healers had had virtually sole responsibility for childbirth and for gynecological problems from the beginnings of recorded history until the 18th century.[31] There are many reasons for the important role of women in medicine during this period. From the Middle Ages on (at least), the female body was thought to be unclean and thus unfit for male healers to treat.[32] Prior to the rise of modern science, medical practice was directed mainly by religious dogma and very little by theory based on empirical observation. Careful study of Plato, Aristotle, Galen, and Christian theology provided the standard training for medical students in the late Middle Ages. Thus women were the only sex familiar with female biology. And, women were by no means restricted to gynecological practice, for they also practiced "general medicine." The story of the takeover of medicine by a small group of males is an account in part of the sheer terrorism of two centuries of witch hunts in which hundreds of thousands of individuals were executed.[33] Over 85 percent of the "witches" were women; many were peasant healers; "symptoms" of witchhood included using "heathen charms" and spells and prescribing medicine without accreditation.[34] In America, Anne Hutchinson, Margaret Jones, and "Mistress Hawkins" are just three of the Massachusetts midwives persecuted as witches.[35] The story of the male takeover of medicine is also in part an account of the introduction of new instruments of medicine, access to which was monopolized first by a few male physicians and then by male physicians as a group. Adrienne Rich describes one of the more lurid of such historical episodes, that in which the introduction of the forceps came to play a significant role in the social process by which men replaced women as attendants on childbirth. Rich reports how three generations of the Chamberlen family kept for nearly a century their "family secret." Their secret was a kit containing a pair of obstetric forceps, a vectis or lever to be used in grasping the back of the head of the fetus, and a fillet or cord used to help in drawing the fetus, once disengaged from an abnormal position, out through the birth-canal.[36] In writing his introduction to a translation of a French text on midwifery, Hugh Chamberlen did not hesitate to remind his readers that the Chamberlens alone possessed "The Secret":

> My Father, Brothers, and myself (tho none other else in Europe as I know) have, by God's Blessing and our Industry, attained to, and long practised a way to deliver women in this case, without any prejudice to them or their infants; tho all others. . . do and must endanger, if not destroy, one or both with hooks.[37]

As Rich points out, Chamberlen's words reveal his willingness to

> sacrifice thousands of women's and children's lives, smugly and complacently, knowing how easily they could be saved, and to justify the withholding of that information in terms of "god's Blessing and our Industry." The men who developed the forceps, symbol of the art of the obstetrician, were profiteers.[38]

When finally, in 1773, the design of the Chamberlen forceps was revealed in Edward Chapman's "Essay for the Improvement of Midwifery," the instrument became "available to all male—and to almost no female—practitioners of the obstetric art."[39] The account of the process by which this occurred, found in both Rich's book and the Ehrenreich and English pamphlet, is well worth reading.

Today witch hunts are not necessary to insure that women know their proper place in health care. Who more naturally could recognize "proper place" in the hospital hierarchy than the lower-middle class women who become RNs?

> RN's occupy an intermediate position in the hospital hierarchy—subordinate to the doctors, but in a supervisory role with respect to practical nurses, aides, and . . . several other kinds of semi-skilled workers. Ideologically, nursing professionalism combines the authoritarianism necessary for the nurse's supervisory role with the authoritarianism, implicit in her relation to the doctors. . . . this sense of mixed status [comes] "naturally" to nurses: RN's are women, they have been socialized to be subordinate to the male doctors. Being of high enough economic class to have afforded nursing education, they can easily feel superior to the aides and practical nurses.[40]

Thus the ideology of professionalism guides higher-level nurses such as RNs to accept the characteristically meritocratic denial of class division in occupational assignment, and to divert the idealized service ethic into a professional "ethic" allowing them to identify "up" with the doctor-managers whose interests, in large part, structure the institution of health care. In this professional ethic, it is not "caring and curing" but institutional loyalty which guides the delivery of health care.

I have been arguing that we can grasp the technology of contemporary nursing only when we see nursing as an industrialized form of "women's work." Let me summarize the features of nursing which also characterize the domestic work from which nursing as an occupation emerged and which today's nurses still perform as their second job.

The labor of the modern family is also characterized by hierarchy and by division of labor. The male is official manager, he is the breadwinner and decision-maker. The female is domestic laborer, performing the repetitive and menial physical labor of family life as well as providing the bulk of the psychological and social services the family requires—the caring and curing of child care and husband-tending, organizing the social life of the family, and so on. Without her labor, he could not spend the time required in training for and performance of his job: his salary actually covers the wages of two workers. For most women of every class, the discrimination and low pay they face in the public labor market make marriage and "family service" look like the most attractive way for them to "earn a living."[41] But the altruistic ethic of service finds perhaps its purest expression in the ideology of women's role in the family—the ideology of the loyal and happy housewife. It makes domestic labor justifiable as a pseudo-career and obscures to outsiders (that is, to husbands and policy-makers) the fact that women's domestic labor is both socially necessary and given virtually no public recognition—not in terms of income, status, or power to determine the conditions of labor.

Furthermore, the ethic of altruism is systematically subverted into an ethic of loyalty to the prevailing structure of the family as an institution and to the husband's interests, right or wrong. This prevents housewives both from identifying and from acting to promote the best interests of their children, of themselves, of the larger community, or, indeed, of their husbands. (I distinguish between men's best interests and their best interests as the dominant culture has defined these. Requiring massive "support forces" at home and dominating others are examples of the latter but not the former.) This subversion of the altruistic ethic into the ethic of loyal wife has been the topic of much recent literature documenting the gruesome details of contemporary domestic life from child-beating, wife-beating, and the high incidence of "mental illness" and depression in married women to the systematic support women provide to the related and inequitable hierarchies of both domestic and political life.[42]

Finally, efforts to "industrialize" domestic labor have been plagued with the same "cooling out" of the service ethic characteristic of the lower echelons of nursing, and for the same reasons. Both privately hired workers, such as maids and house cleaners, and publicly hired workers, such as those in many of the new day-care centers, are paid so little and given so little power over the conditions of their labor that it requires what can only be seen as an almost fanatic dose of altruism for them to continue to identify and serve the real needs of their "clients" or charges. In many cases, they understandably come to regard their industrialized domestic labor as "just a job." The exceptions to this rule are significant. Only community-organized domestic labor—whether in parent-run nurseries or, more broadly, in some of the communal living groups—has succeeded in industrializing domestic labor and yet maintaining the service ethic. In these cases the new ways of organizing labor were selected with an interest in maximizing desirable social relations as defined by the workers.

It seems characteristic of "women's work"—whether at home or in the "helping professions"—that it is technologized not to suit the needs of the women working or of their "charges," but to serve the interests of other powerful groups in society from which women are systematically excluded.

What are these "other groups" whose interests have in fact shaped contemporary health care? Three forces have been dominant since the end of the Second World War. These are the academic medical empires, the health-care financiers, and the health-care profiteers.[43] Their interests are not always identical with the interests of the recipients of health-care patients—nor with the interests of health-care workers. Sometimes the interests of the decision-makers actually conflict with patients' and nurses' interests.

Research and education are the main interests of the academic medical establishment. The academicians

> contributed to the scientific and technological advances in medicine following World War II. However they gained their dominant position in the health-care delivery system not because of the scientific and technical advances, but because they used the prestige from federal research grants to insure plenty of paying patients to fill their beds.[44]

Often the interests of the academic establishment support good health care. Because of basic research, antibiotics were discovered and they contributed greatly to human health. However, there are many cases where the interests of the medical academy conflict with the interests of patients. The overriding desire for experimental results can lead to the use of inadequately tested drugs on patients; hospitals are often organized into many specialty clinics which further the education of medical students and the interests of researchers but which frequently result in confused, discouraged, and sometimes mistreated patients.[45]

The largest of the private financiers of health care is Blue Cross. However, Blue Cross was initially organized by hospitals, and it pays only for health care delivered in hospitals even though the concentration of health care in hospitals does not always maximize benefits to patients. Two sorts of objections may be raised to restricting the delivery of health care to hospitals. In the first place, the concentration of medical resources in hospitals makes these resources less available to patients under some conditions; and, secondly, some kinds of health "problems" (impending death, childbirth, and chronic illness) are accompanied by emotional and physical needs better served at home.[46]

Finally, the third force shaping contemporary health care is the health profiteers. Hospital supply companies and drug companies in particular have reaped huge profits from scientific discoveries, profits paid for by patients; and, furthermore, they have contributed to the concentration of health care in hospitals.[47]

Thus the nature and structure of nursing have in effect been the consequences of the ability of these three groups of policy-makers to translate their interests into practice. The ability of nurses to care and cure is limited by the power of these three forces to determine which of the alternative technologies of health care will be brought into existence.[48] None of these policy-makers has an interest in giving greater control over working conditions to health-care workers, and none has caring and curing as his highest priority.

CONCLUSION

I have been arguing that technology is not an autonomous social force providing its own ends, nor are particular technologies value-neutral means to ends which are chosen entirely in the moral/political arena. Instead, technological decisions are decisions about how to organize human labor. Thus they are in part moral/political decisions, though only *some* technological alternatives are compatible with any given moral/political goal. The causal influences go in both directions. Moral/political values influence decisions to develop better ways of organizing labor as well as choices among available alternative technologies; but, also, the ways in which labor is organized can support or undermine a prevailing moral/political system or a desired moral/political goal.

The structure of health care has been a case in point. The history of medicine reveals many places where moral/political goals shaped both the development of instruments and machines and the way the labor of health care has been organized. It should not surprise us to find that nursing, traditionally marked as a woman's occupation, has been structured by the moral/political forces which have shaped women's lives more generally. For those interested in improving the quality of health care and the nature of contemporary nursing, this is cause for both pessimism and optimism. Because of the isomorphism between the structure of health care and the structure of social life, attempts to institute fairer and more adequate technologies of health care can expect to meet all the resistance raised in opposition to attempts to bring about fairer and more adequate institutions in society in general. But, on the other hand, when democratizing winds of change touch health care, they also cut deeply into oppressive aspects of the moral/political climate of our society in general.[49]

We all have an interest in restructuring health care so that the special interests of a few groups are not allowed to override our general social needs. Thus we all have an interest in joining nurses in critically examining the political and social forces which shape the technological decisions in health care.

NOTES

1. As quoted by Bernard Gendron, *Technology and the Human Condition*, New York: St. Martin's Press, 1977, pp. 11-12.

2. *Ibid.*, p. 4.

3. *Ibid.*, p. 90.

4. For an illuminating critical analysis of the idea that technology is an auton-

omous force, see Langdon Winner, *Autonomous Technology*, Cambridge: MIT Press, 1977.

5. Cf. Winner's useful distinction between technology as apparatus, as technique, and as organization, *op. cit.*, pp. 11-12. All three are involved in any given "technological alternative," as I argue below.

6. Stanley Joel Reiser, "Therapeutic Choice and Moral Doubt in a Technological Age," *Doing Better and Feeling Worse*, (ed.) J.H. Knowles, New York: W.W. Norton, 1977, p. 47.

7. Walsh McDermott, "Evaluating the Physician and His Technology," *Doing Better and Feeling Worse*, (ed.) J.H. Knowles, New York: W.W. Norton, 1977, p. 143.

8. For a discussion of the problem with respect to the physical and the social sciences, see my "Does Objectivity in Social Science Require Value-Neutrality?" *Soundings*, LX, 1977, and "Four Contributions Values Can Make to the Objectivity of Social Science," *PSA 1978 Vol. I*, (eds.) Peter Asquith and Ian Hacking, East Lansing: Philosophy of Science Association, 1978.

9. Edgar Zilsel, "The Sociological Roots of Science," *American Journal of Sociology* (1942). Reprinted in *Science, Technology and Freedom*, (eds.) W. Truitt and R. Solomons, New York: Houghton Mifflin, 1974, p. 88.

10. Barbara Ehrenreich and Deirdre English, "The Manufacture of Housework," *Socialist Revolution* 26 (1975). Ruth Schwartz Cowan, "Two Washes in the Morning and a Bridge Party at Night: The American Housewife Between the Wars," *Women's Studies* 3 (1976).

11. Cf. Willis Truitt and R. Solomons, in *Science, Technology and Freedom*, (eds.) W. Truitt and R. Solomons, New York: Houghton Mifflin, 1974; J.D. Bernal, "Marx and Science," in the same volume; José Ortega y Gasset, "Thoughts on Technology," in *Philosophy and Technology*, (eds.) C. Mitcham and R. Mackay, New York: The Free Press, 1972; Ernst Junger, "Technology as the Mobilization of the World through the Gestalt of the Worker," in the same volume; C.B. Macpherson, "Democratic Theory: Ontology and Technology," in the same volume.

12. For accounts of why women cluster in the helping professions and of the history of the emergence of the helping professions, see Margaret Adams, "The Compassion Trap," in *Woman in Sexist Society*, (eds.) V. Gornick and B. Moran, New York: Basic Books, 1971; Susan Reverby, "Health: Women's Work," in *Prognosis Negative: Crisis in the Health Care System*, (ed.) D. Kotelchuck, New York: Random House, 1976; and Eli Zaretsky, *Capitalism, The Family and Personal Life*, New York: Harper and Row, 1976.

13. Barbara Caress, "The Health Workforce: Bigger Pie, Smaller Pieces," *Prognosis Negative: Crisis in the Health Care System*, (ed.) D. Kotelchuck, New York: Random House, 1976, p. 169; Ivan L. Bennett, Jr., "Technology as a Shaping Force," in *Doing Better and Feeling Worse*, (ed.) J.H. Knowles, New York: W.W. Norton, 1977, p. 126.

14. John and Barbara Ehrenreich, "Hospital Workers: A Case Study in the 'New Working Class,'" *Prognosis Negative: Crisis in the Health Care System*, (ed.) D. Kotelchuck, New York: Random House, 1976, p. 186.

15. Caress, p. 168.

16. Ehrenreich, *op. cit.*, p. 188.

17. *Ibid.*, pp. 187-188.

18. *Ibid.*, p. 188.

19. Quoted in Reverby, *op. cit.*, p. 176.

20. *Ibid.*, p. 175.

21. *Ibid.*

22. Ehrenreich, *op. cit.*, p. 189.

23. *Ibid.*, p. 191.

24. *Ibid.*, p. 192.

25. *Ibid.*, p. 191.

26. Quoted in Thomas L. Haskell, "Power to the Experts," *The New York Review* XXIV, Oct. 13, 1977, p. 28.

27. Ehrenreich, *op. cit.*, p. 193.

28. *Ibid.*

29. Burton J. Bledstein, *The Culture of Professionalism: The Middle Class and the Development of Higher Education in America*, New York: Norton, 1977. I have critically examined the ideal of a meritocracy in "Equality of Opportunity, Meritocracy, and the Democratic Ethic," *Philosophical Forum*, X(1979).

30. Ehrenreich, *op. cit.*, p. 195.

31. Adrienne Rich, *Of Woman Born*, New York: W.W. Norton, 1976, p. 131.

32. *Ibid.*, p. 134.

33. Barbara Ehrenreich and Deirdre English, *Witches, Midwives and Nurses: A History of Women Healers*, New York: The Feminist Press, 1973, p. 8.

34. Rich, *op. cit.*, p. 135.

35. Rich, *op. cit.*, p. 135.

36. Rich, *op. cit.*, p. 143.

37. *Ibid.*, p. 144.

38. *Ibid.*

39. *Ibid.*, p. 145.

40. Ehrenreich, *op. cit.*, p. 195.

41. Francine D. Blau, "Women in the Labor Force: An Overview," in *Women: A Feminist Perspective*, (ed.) Jo Freeman, Palo Alto: Mayfield, 1975.

42. Pauline Bart, "Depression in Middle-Aged Women"; in *Woman in Sexist Society*, (eds.) V. Gornick and B. Moran, New York: Basic Books, 1971; Jessie Bernard, "The Paradox of the Happy Marriage," in the same volume; Dair Gillespie, "Who Has the Power? The Marital Struggle," *Journal of Marriage and the Family*, 1971.

43. David Kotelchuck, "The Health-Care Delivery System," in *Prognosis Negative: Crisis in the Health Care System*, (ed.) Kotelchuck, New York: Random House, 1976, p. 2.

44. *Ibid.*

45. *Ibid.*

46. *Ibid.*

47. *Ibid.*

48. A valuable discussion of obstacles to change in health care is Robert R. Alford's *Health Care Politics: Ideological and Interest Group Barriers to Reform*, Chicago: University of Chicago Press, 1975.

49. Ehrenreich and Ehrenreich agree, *op. cit.*, p. 199ff.

BIBLIOGRAPHY

Adams, Margaret. "The Compassion Trap," *Woman in Sexist Society*, (eds.) V. Gornick and B. Moran, New York: Basic Books, 1971.

Alford, Robert R. *Health Care Politics: Ideological and Interest Group Barriers to Reform*, Chicago: University of Chicago Press, 1977.

Barker-Benfield, Ben. "The Spermatic Economy: A Nineteenth Century View of Sexuality," *Feminist Studies*, 1:1, Summer 1972.

Bart, Pauline B. "Depression in Middle-Aged Women," *Woman in Sexist Society*, (eds.) V. Gornick and B. Moran, New York: Basic Books, 1971.

Bennett, Jr., Ivan L. "Technology as a Shaping Force," *Doing Better and Feeling Worse*, (ed.) J. H. Knowles, New York: W. W. Norton, 1977.

Bernal, J.D. "Marx and Science," in *Science, Technology, and Freedom*, (eds.) Truitt and Solomons, New York: Houghton Mifflin, 1974.

Bernard, Jessie. "The Paradox of the Happy Marriage." *Woman in Sexist Society*, (eds.) V. Gornick and B. Moran, New York: Basic Books, 1971.

Blau, Francine D. "Women in the Labor Force: An Overview," *Women: A Feminist Perspective*, (ed.) J. Freeman, Palo Alto: Mayfield, 1975.

Bledstein, Burton J. *The Culture of Professionalism: The Middle Class and the Development of Higher Education in America*, New York: Norton, 1977.

Caress, Barbara. "The Health Workforce: Bigger Pie, Smaller Pieces," *Prognosis Negative: Crisis in the Health Care System*, (ed.) D. Kotelchuck, New York: Random House, 1976.

Cowan, Ruth Schwartz. "Two Washes in the Morning and a Bridge Party at Night: The American Housewife Between the Wars," *Women's Studies*, 3, 1976.

Ehrenreich, Barbara, and Deirdre English. *Witches, Midwives and Nurses: A History of Women Healers*, New York: The Feminist Press, 1973.

Ehrenreich, Barbara, and Deidre English. "The Manufacture of Housework," *Socialist Revolution*, 26, 1975.

Ehrenreich, John and Barbara. "Hospital Workers: A Case Study in the 'New Working Class.'" *Prognosis Negative: Crisis in the Health Care System*, (ed.) D. Kotelchuck, New York: Random House, 1976.

Gendron, Bernard. *Technology and the Human Condition*, New York: St. Martin's Press, 1977.

Gillespie, Dair. "Who Has the Power? The Marital Struggle," *Journal of Marriage and the Family*, 1971.

Harding, Sandra. "Does Objectivity in Social Science Require Value-Neutrality?" *Soundings*, LX, 1977.

_____. "Four Contributions Values Can Make to the Objectivity of Social Science," *PSA 1978 Vol. I*, (eds.) Peter Asquith and Ian Hacking, East Lansing: Philosophy of Science Association, 1978.

_____. "Is the Equality of Opportunity Principle Democratic?" *Philosophical Forum*, X, 1979.

Haskell, Thomas L. "Power to the Experts," *The New York Review* XXIV, October 13, 1977. (A review of Bledstein's book).

Junger, Ernst. "Technology as the Mobilization of the World through the Gestalt of the Worker," in *Philosophy and Technology*, (eds.) C. Mitcham and R. Mackey, New York: The Free Press, 1972.

Knowles, John H. "The Responsibility of the Individual," *Doing Better and Feeling Worse*, (ed.) J. H. Knowles, New York: W. W. Norton, 1977.

Kobrin, Frances E. "The American Midwife Controversy: A Crisis of Professionalization," *Bulletin of the History of Medicine*, July-August, 1966.

Kotelchuck, David. "The Health-Care Delivery System," *Prognosis Negative: Crisis in the Health Care System*, (ed.) D. Kotelchuck, New York: Random House, 1976.

Macpherson, C. B. "Democratic Theory: Ontology and Technology," in *Philosophy and Technology*, (eds.) C. Mitcham and R. Mackey, New York: The Free Press, 1972.

McDermott, Walsh. "Evaluating the Physician and His Technology," *Doing Better and Feeling Worse*, (ed.) J. H. Knowles, New York: W. W. Norton, 1977.

Ortega y Gasset, José. "Thoughts on Technology," in *Philosophy and Technology*, (eds.) C. Mitcham and R. Mackey, New York: The Free Press, 1972.

Reiser, Stanley Joel. "Therapeutic Choice and Moral Doubt in a Technological Age," *Doing Better and Feeling Worse*, (ed.) J. H. Knowles, New York: W. W. Norton, 1977.

Reverby, Susan. "Health: Women's Work." *Prognosis Negative: Crisis in the Health Care System*, (ed.) D. Kotelchuck, New York: Random House, 1976.

Rich, Adrienne. *Of Woman Born*, New York: W. W. Norton, 1976.

Spieler, Emily. "Division of Laborers," *Prognosis Negative: Crisis in the Health Care System*, (ed.) D. Kotelchuck, New York: Random House, 1976.

Szasz, Thomas, "The Witch as Healer," in *The Manufacture of Madness*, New York: Delta Books, 1971.

Thomas, Lewis. "On the Science and Technology of Medicine," *Doing Better and Feeling Worse*, (ed.) J. H. Knowles, New York: W. W. Norton, 1977.

Truitt, W. and R. Solomons. *Science, Technology and Freedom*, New York: Houghton Mifflin, 1974.

Winner, Langdon. *Autonomous Technology*, Cambridge: MIT Press, 1977.

Zaretsky, Eli. *Capitalism, The Family and Private Life*, New York: Harper and Row, 1976.

Zilsel, Edgar. "The Sociological Roots of Science." *American Journal of Sociology*, January, 1942. Reprinted in *Science, Technology and Freedom*, (eds.) W. Truitt and R. Solomons, New York: Houghton Mifflin, 1974.

Part II

IDEALS OF NURSING: PHILOSOPHICAL DIMENSIONS OF NURSING PRACTICE

4

Existential Advocacy: Philosophical Foundation of Nursing*

Sally Gadow

INTRODUCTION: AGAINST META-NURSING

Turning points occur in the history of a profession when radical questioning and clarification of major tenets become essential for further growth. We recognize such a turning point now in nursing. The direction in which nursing develops will determine whether the profession draws closer to the medical model, with its commitment to science, technology, and cure; reverts to historical nursing models, with their essentially intuitive approaches; or creates a new philosophy that sets contemporary nursing distinctively apart from both traditional nursing and modern medicine.

However, the question of whether such a distinctive concept of nursing is possible has not yet been resolved. One sociologist suggests that, rather than the evolution of a new philosophy of nursing, nurses

*Appreciation is expressed to Ann Davis, H. Tristram Engelhardt, Jr., Elizabeth Maloney, Teresa Stanley, and J. Melvin Woody, whose extensive and thoughtful commentaries on the paper as originally presented have contributed significantly to its revision.

will evolve out of nursing: "nursing will still be nursing, but it will be carried on by persons of other occupational affiliations."[1] What will nurses be doing while someone else is doing the nursing? They will be moving on to meta-nursing. In the words of one of them, "The role of the nurse must be transcended in order to relate as human being to human being."[2]

If nursing is conceptualized in such a way that it must be transcended in order to involve the nurse as a human being, it is not surprising that nurses relinquish some of their functions to other health workers. Nevertheless, the fact that they still consider themselves nurses suggests that the meta-nursing to which they turn is *not* a transcending or outgrowing of nursing, but an early expression, not yet explicit, of new possibilities within nursing.

This phenomenon, that persons who have moved beyond nursing still consider themselves nurses, reflects the belief which is the premise of this chapter—that nursing ought to be defined philosophically rather than sociologically, that is, defined by the ideal nature and purpose of the nurse-patient relation rather than by a specific set of behaviors. When the concept of nursing is addressed as a philosophical ideal rather than as an empirical construct, we see immediately that it is contradictory to speak of nurses transcending nursing or delegating it to non-nurses. In other words, if nursing is distinguished by its *philosophy* of care and not by its care *functions*, and if nurses themselves formulate that philosophy, they transcend a particular concept of nursing only in order to realize a more developed concept, an ideal: a philosophy of nursing which unifies and enhances the experience of the individuals involved rather than devaluing and alienating that experience.

Some of the definitions of an ideal concept of nursing are familiar to anyone acquainted with the history of nursing: the nurse as healer, champion of the sick poor, parent-surrogate, physician-surrogate, contracted clinician, personal counselor, and health educator. The concept that I will propose as the philosophical foundation and ideal of nursing is that of advocacy—not the concept of advocacy implied in the patients' rights movement, in which any health professional is potentially a consumer advocate, but a fundamental, existential advocacy for which the nurse alone, among all the health professionals, is uniquely suited, and which is as distinct from consumer advocacy as it is from paternalism.

This concept of existential advocacy is not simply another alternative in the list of past and present concepts of nursing, nor does it imply a rejection of all other concepts. Rather, it is proposed as the philosophical foundation upon which the patient and the nurse can freely decide whether their relation shall be that of child and parent, client and counselor, friend and friend, colleague and colleague, and so on through the range of possibilities.

In order to elaborate this proposed ideal of existential advocacy, I will first distinguish it from paternalism and from patient's rights advocacy. I will then describe advocacy nursing as a resolution of two conflicts within health care that manifest in nursing the greatest urgency as well as the greatest possibility for solution: (1) the dichotomy between the personal and the professional involvement of the nurse, and (2) the discrepancy between the lived body and the object body of the patient. Finally, I will propose that existential advocacy as the essence of nursing is the nurse's participation with the patient in determining the unique meaning which the experience of health, illness, suffering, or dying is to have for that individual.

CONCEPTUAL FRAMEWORK

The conflict between advocacy and paternalism is felt most acutely by the nurse, since it is the nurse who must reconcile nursing's traditional alliance with the patient and the modern allegiance to medicine. Moreover, humanistic and authoritarian tendencies compete in nursing with particular intensity because of the comprehensive, yet personal, nature of nursing care. The nurse attends the patient as a whole, not just as a single problem or system. The nurse attends the patient during periods of sustained contact, and often provides the mundane intimacies usually considered to be self-care. Thus the nurse is in the ideal position among health-care providers to experience the patient as a unique human being with individual strengths and complexities—a precondition for advocacy. On the other hand, the potential for paternalism is as great as that for advocacy, for just those reasons. The comprehensiveness, immediacy, and continuity of care present an exceptional opportunity for powerful influence over individuals—the precondition for paternalism.

Paternalism

The concept of advocacy proposed here is in essence the opposite of paternalism. For that reason, it is important to formulate clearly the meaning of paternalism which is being used.

Paternalistic acts and attitudes are those that limit the liberty or rights of individuals for their own interest. Paternalism implies the existence of coercion, since the individuals who voluntarily submit to a restriction are theoretically exercising their liberty in the making of choice. A more explicit meaning of paternalism, then, is the use of coercion in order to provide a good that is not desired by the one whom it is intended to benefit.[3] Such a formulation deliberately leaves open whether the person refuses the "good" because it is not recognized as a good, or because its value is lower than other goods in the person's hierarchy of values. For example, the refusal of blood transfusions by Jehovah's Witness patients may not reflect the failure to judge health or life to be a good, but the judging of another end to have a higher value. In either case, interference in that decision is paternalistic.

It has been argued that the essential element in paternalism (other than its motivation, the intent to obtain a good for the person affected) is not coercion, but "the violation of moral rules."[4] But this view fails to account for the case, for example, in which a woman anticipating the discovery of a malignancy asks that she not be told if her fears are confirmed, and the physician complies by lying to her. Here a moral rule has been violated in the interest of the person affected, but it is doubtful whether the authors of this view would judge the action paternalistic. On the contrary, overriding the patient's wishes and forcing the truth upon her (if done for her own good) would count as paternalism.[5] The single moral "rule," then, which is negated by paternalism is the prohibition against coercion, here defined as the forcing of individuals either to act in some way that is contrary to their wishes or to submit to someone else's action which is contrary to their wishes. An example of the former is the requirement that even unwilling students must write examinations; of the latter, the insistence that uncooperative patients submit to any diagnostic procedures that the practitioner believes necessary.

In summary, there are two principal elements in paternalism: (1) the intent—obtaining what is believed to be a good for the other person, and (2) the effect—violating the person's known wishes in the matter.

The meaning of paternalism is formulated differently by its defenders—not in terms of violation but of assistance. This view expresses the belief that in matters affecting an individual's well-being, the person's decisions should be made by those most capable of knowing what actions are in the person's interest.[6] Accordingly, it is inherent in professional responsibility always to act in the patient's interest. Paternalism is not a violation of the patient's right of self-determination so much as it is a protection of the patient's right to the best possible care that can be given.

However, this positive interpretation of paternalism only confuses matters, since it reduces paternalism to an identity with an equally simplistic meaning of advocacy, that is, acting on behalf of another. With this confusion, the most paternalistic professional can claim to be the staunchest patient advocate. Indeed, paternalism becomes the most thoroughgoing form of advocacy, inasmuch as it goes the length of even opposing patients' wishes in order to act in their interest. The conflation of paternalism and advocacy is a confusion which negates the truth of both, namely, that paternalism is a violation of the right of self-determination, and that advocacy does not consist in acting for another. The two are philosophically opposing concepts.

Patient's Rights and Consumerism

If advocacy and paternalism are opposites, and paternalism is the patient's submission to the professional's wishes, does this mean that advocacy limits the professional's actions to whatever the patient wishes? Is advocacy a form of consumer protection, in which the role of the professional is only to provide information necessary for the patient's selection among available courses of action? Is the advocate nurse a technical advisor whose responsibility stops short of recommending one option over another, lest that recommendation become coercion?

The answer to these is no, for professional consumerism would only seem to be a sophisticated form of paternalism, which insists that, in the interest of individuals' autonomy, they be forced to make important decisions alone, with only technical assistance. The fact that information which was traditionally denied to patients is now provided does not alter the paternalistic assumption that that is *all* that should be provided in order for patients to act autonomously, nor, for that matter, the assumption that individuals ought to act autonomously.

The current concept of patients' rights advocacy should be understood in this light, as a part of the wider movement of consumerism. "Patient advocacy is seeing that the patient knows what to expect and what is his right to have, and then displaying the willingness and courage to see that our system does not prevent his getting it."[7] From this point of view, the advocate is, at best, a troubleshooter willing to intervene when the system violates an individual's rights.[8]

Advocacy

The concept of advocacy (from this point on the term "advocacy" will be used to mean existential advocacy) is distinct from both paternalism and consumer protection. It is based upon the principle that freedom of self-determination is the most fundamental and valuable human right.

In negative terms, this implies that the right of self-determination ought not to be infringed upon even in the interest of health. The professional, while obligated to act in the patient's interest, is not permitted to define that interest in any way contrary to the patient's definition: it is not the professional but the patient who determines what "best interest" shall mean.

In positive terms, this meaning of advocacy has far greater implications for the professional and extends beyond the narrow realm of proscriptions into the realm of ideals. The ideal which existential advocacy expresses is this: that individuals be *assisted* by nursing to *authentically* exercise their freedom of self-determination. By authentic is meant a way of reaching decisions which are truly one's own—decisions that express all that one believes important about oneself and the world, the entire complexity of one's values.

Individuals can express their wholeness and uniqueness as valuing beings only if their full complexity of values—including contradictions and conflicts—is clearly in mind, having been reexamined and clarified in the new context. Yet, that clarification is the most difficult precisely when it is most needed, when a situation arises which threatens to overturn previously stable values. In such situations, of which health impairment is a paradigm, individuals face the necessity of either recreating their values or recreating their situation according to their existing hierarchy of values. The paternalistic response to this is simple: never mind examining values, because health is the highest human value. The response of consumerism to the patient is still more simple: once you have been informed of all of your options, do whatever you like.

The response of advocacy differs from both of these. It is not based on an assumption about what individuals *should want* to do, nor does it consist in protecting individuals' *rights* to do what they want. It is the effort to help persons *become clear about what they want* to do, by helping them discern and clarify their values in the situation, and on the basis of that self-examination, to reach decisions which express their reaffirmed, perhaps recreated, complex of values. Only in this way, when the valuing self is engaged and expressed in its entirety, can a person's decision be actually *self*-determined instead of being a decision which is not determined by others. [9]

ADVOCACY AND CONTRADICTIONS IN THE NURSE-PATIENT RELATION

Two basic discrepancies in health care prevent authentic self-determination, despite the lip service paid to "patient autonomy." They are first the dichotomy between personal and professional involvement of the practitioner, and second, that between the lived body and the object body of the patient. Because both of these conflicts result in fragmentation of the patient as well as the practitioner, their effect is to seriously limit the extent of the person that is involved in making decisions. If nursing is to accomplish its purpose in existential advocacy—i.e., if patients are to be assisted in making decisions which are genuinely their own because they fully express their own reaffirmed or recreated values—then nursing must resolve both of these discrepancies. As long as either remains, a source of self-alienation and personal disunity, the patient is effectively prevented from exercising his or her right of self-determination.

Personal versus Professional

The movement of humanistic health care has attempted to soften the distinction between the person and the professional. Professionals are encouraged to become involved with and attentive to patients as individuals—in other words, to behave more like persons than just professionals—while patients have begun to assume some of the responsibilities formerly reserved for the professional.

But the dichotomy persists, nevertheless. In all health professions, new practitioners are warned that becoming personally involved with patients is unprofessional (in spite of patients' complaints that their care is too impersonal). The traditional view maintains that the personal and the professional are mutually exclusive aspects of the practitioner: behaving professionally entails the avoidance of any personal interactions; i.e., behavior expressing the professional's feelings, values, or idiosyncracies. From this point of view, individuals are interchangeable, because none of their individuality is allowed into their interactions with patients.

Another version of this view considers the professional role to be one among the many in which the person engages. Different elements of the person are distributed among the various roles, with the result that at least something of the individual is expressed in professional behavior. That "something," however, usually includes at most the person's scientific, technical, and managerial capabilities; the emotional, esthetic, and contemplative, among others, are confined to other domains of the person's life.

Both of these views have the inevitable effect of fragmenting the individual, in this case the nurse, who guards against any "leaking" of the personal domains into the professional. Because of that exclusion of significant elements of the person from the professional relation, self-estrangement occurs within the nurse and, consequently, within the patient. Regarding the *patient* as a "whole" would seem to require nothing less than the *nurse* acting as a "whole" person. Therefore, the nurse who withholds parts of the self is unlikely to allow the patient to emerge as a whole, or to comprehend that wholeness if it does emerge.

Are we justified in assuming that the traditional view is right, that one essential feature of "professional" is its exclusion of the personal? In different terms, does the introduction of the personal into the professional domain so alter the nature of "professional" that its distinctiveness disappears and it becomes essentially no different from giving help to a friend or to oneself?

To answer, we can examine, phenomenologically, the differences between patient and professional in a hypothetical situation—for example, the relation between two women who are professional colleagues, one of whom provides nursing care for the other. In such a relation between professional equals, any nonessential differences (such as expertise) disappear, and it should be possible to discern only essential differences. To further avoid confusion with nonessential differences, we can stipulate that the colleague designated as the care provider suffers from the same disease as the person receiving care. Here, the two persons relating to one another as patient and nurse have a comparable understanding of the health problem in question— there is no difference in their competence to deal with the disease as a clinical entity. However, the essential differences arise with respect to their dealing with the illness as a personal experience. Those differences can be classified in terms of (1) focus, (2) intensity, and (3) perspective.

(1) The focus of the patient is directed to the problem at hand and its effect upon her life; her concern is unavoidably self-oriented. In contrast, the focus of the professional is directed away from herself toward the other. Her feelings of distress over the other's pain may be expressed, but not in order to obtain either relief or help from the

patient. There is not, as in personal relations, a mutuality in which both are equally concerned about the other (with each one also maintaining some degree of self-interest). In the professional relation, the practitioner is interested in the other's good more than in her own, while the patient is concerned primarily about her well-being rather than the other's.

Personal relations too, though fundamentally relations of mutuality, can assume a one-directional focus when one of the persons is in distress, but two important differences remain between that situation and the professional relation. In friendship, mutuality is the accepted ideal, and departures from it, when one or the other person needs unusual attention, are understood to be temporary. The basis of the professional relation is the established disposition of one of the persons to attend to the other without receiving attention in return. Furthermore, in personal relations, because of the ideal of mutuality, there is a point beyond which a one-sided focus becomes unacceptable, and the relation must either return to a reciprocal one or dissolve. In the professional relation, such a limit does not exist, inasmuch as the professional does not depend upon receiving the attention of the patient to make the relationship worthwhile.

(2) The intensity of the situation is experienced differently by the professional and the patient. The latter is caught up in the immediacy of her distress, the urgency of the symptoms as compelling phenomena in themselves. The professional may feel the same intensity, particularly when she has experienced the symptoms herself, but she is not bound by their immediacy. Her continued focus upon the patient makes the professional remain at the level of reflection rather than feeling. This is in order to integrate feelings and knowledge in the attempt to alleviate the patient's distress, and thereby free her from the limits of immediacy. Thus it is the form and direction, not the degree, of intensity which necessarily differ in the two persons.

This difference in intensity can occur in personal relations as well, but, like the one-sided focus described in (1), it is a departure from the ideal of mutuality, in which the intensity of one's experience is fully shared by the other in its immediacy before becoming the object of reflection. In the professional relation, the intensity felt by the nurse is not a sharing with the patient which has value in itself, value that is independent of helping the other. Rather, the intensity serves as an intensification of the reflective process necessary for help to be given. Being able to help has greater value than simply sharing the other's experience, an inversion of the values—sharing and helping—in personal relations.

(3) In addition to differences in focus and intensity, the perspectives of the two persons differ. The professional is "externally" involved, despite the similarities between herself and the patient, whereas the patient is involved in a radically interior way, feeling the pain "from the inside" and knowing that, although others may have the same disease, it is only *her* body which is affected in this instance.

This is the difference usually designated as the nurse's objectivity and the patient's subjectivity. Unfortunately, these terms are often used specifically to indicate degrees of emotional involvement. The implication there is that the essential difference in the two persons' perspectives is that the patient is more and the nurse less emotional. This ignores the possibility that both persons might experience emotional intensity, even though, in the professional, that intensity does not remain at the level of immediacy, but acts as an intensification of other dimensions of the person.

The essential difference in the perspectives of the two persons is related, not to emotion, but to the body. Only the patient can experience her body as an interiority, a living subjectivity, and only someone other than the patient can experience her body as a technical object, a thing to be regarded strictly scientifically.

Because patient and nurse have fundamentally different modes of access to the patient's body, and thus experience it in opposite ways, their understanding of it differs. The patient understands her body as a unique reality that cannot be expressed through types or generalizations. The nurse understands the patient's body as a part of the world of objects, and therefore, most effectively approached through clinical categories. She is, of course, ultimately concerned with the patient as a unique human being, but she addresses the body's phenomena as instances of general types of phenomena. "Pain here" is categorized as "gastralgia," for example, in order to apply the appropriate remedy. In short, in their involvement with the patient's body, the patient is oriented toward uniqueness, the professional toward typification.

The patient herself, as a professional whose involvement with patients' bodies is characteristically oriented toward the general, can, to some extent, combine the general with the unique in considering her own body. But because both approaches are required in ideal health care, each one needs to be developed as fully as possible, and this the person cannot do alone, even in her dual role as patient and professional. The two orientations, though complementary, are categorically different and, in most cases, the patient engages only in one by diminishing her engagement in the other. For the two perspectives to be thoroughly utilized together, a second person is needed to develop the objective dimension.

Again, the question arises whether the second person need be a professional, or could as well be a friend. Here, as in the differences in focus and intensity, the value of mutuality in personal relations prevents the friend from maintaining a one-sided approach, except as a temporary departure from supporting the other as an ultimately indivisible unity of subject and object. The professional, unlike the friend or the patient herself, is able to maintain for the patient the one perspective toward her experience which is the most difficult for her to develop: sustained objectivity.

In considering these three differences between personal and professional relations and between the patient and the professional, we see that the most commonly assumed difference is absent: the nurse does not manifest less involvement as a person than does the patient or the friend. On the contrary, the differences described above suggest that, while the form and direction of involvement differ significantly, the "amount" of the person involved is equally great.

On this basis, a solution to the personal/professional dichotomy can be proposed in the following way. Professional involvement is not an *alternative* to other kinds of involvement, such as emotional, esthetic, physical, or intellectual. It is a deliberate synthesis of all of these, a participation of the *entire* self, using every dimension of the person as resource in the professional relation.

This concept of professional involvement, as a unifying and directing of one's entire self in relation to another's need, is entailed by the concept of existential advocacy. Advocacy implies that patients can be assisted in reaching decisions which express their complex totality as individuals only by nurses who themselves act out of the same explicit self-unity, allowing no dimension of themselves to be exempt from the professional relation. Furthermore, the nurse, among the health professionals, is uniquely able to actualize such a holistic view of the professional. Nursing care, because of its immediate, sustained, and often intimate nature, as well as its scientific and ethical complexity, offers ready avenues for every dimension of the professional to be engaged, including the emotional, rational, esthetic, intuitive, physical, and philosophical.

One objection is commonly raised against resolving the personal/professional dichotomy in this way. It is that the professional's emotional involvement entails, for the patient, the risk of biased clinical judgment, and for the professional, the risk of personal suffering and emotional depletion. Such an objection, however, is based on a seriously limited view of emotional involvement. It assumes that through the feeling of another's suffering, "suffering itself becomes infectious."[10] In other words, to participate in another's emotion and have direct knowledge of it is to experience that emotion oneself and be as bound by its immediacy as the person who is actually experiencing it.

A significantly different possibility for emotional involvement, which that view does not consider, is the experience of "fellow-feeling" described by Max Scheler. Fellow-feeling is distinct from emotional infection and from merely perceiving the other's emotion. "It is indeed a case of *feeling* the other's feeling, not just knowing it, nor judging that the other has it; but it is not the same as going through the experience itself."[11]

The distinction between fellow-feeling and emotional infection, or identification, reflects the same difference described earlier in relation to the different focus and intensity of patient and professional. The focus of fellow-feeling is the *other's* feeling, not one's own, which prevents emotional participation from becoming infectious identification. The emotion of the patient is not merely reproduced or reenacted within the professional (making the latter the one needing help). Rather, the patient's feeling is "vicariously visualized" in order to make possible a *"directing* of feeling towards the other's joy or suffering."[12] To participate in the suffering of the other in fact precludes the professional's suffering in herself, since it is then her own experience, not the patient's, which would be the object of her focus.

The difference of intensity is related to this difference of focus. In fellow-feeling, in contrast to emotional identification (i.e., in the professional's feeling as distinct from the patient's), the intensity is consciously directed, whereas in the experiencing of one's own emotion or the identification with another's, involvement is immediate rather than directed, involuntary rather than deliberate, and often unconscious. It is the failure to distinguish this different intensity of fellow-feeling from emotional identification which gives rise to the objection that emotional involvement distorts professional judgment. In emotional infection the nurse indeed succumbs to the same involuntary and unconscious immediacy which the patient experiences, and it could be argued that that use of intensity might well distort judgment. But fellow-feeling is a different, *directed* intensity, "a genuine *outreaching* and entry into the other person and his individual situation, a true and authentic transcendence of one's self."[13]

Fellow-feeling is but one example of the concrete solutions possible in advocacy nursing: resolution of the personal/professional dichotomy, in this case by the nurse's deliberate emotional participation with the patient. For the patient's emotional complexity to be understood and supported, the emotional dimension of the nurse's own being cannot be excluded, but must be consciously and directly engaged. Moreover, just as with the emotional, so too with the esthetic, intuitive, physical, philosophical, and all other dimensions of personal reality can and must be brought to bear as essential, positive elements in the professional relation.[14] The absolute prerequisite for advocacy— advocating the patient's own individually created values—is the participation of the advocate as an individual, a complete unity unfragmented by exclusion of any part of the self.

Lived Body versus Object Body

The nurse's dichotomy—between personal and professional involvement—is directly related to the patient's dichotomy—between the body as a private, lived reality and a public object open to inspection.

The nurse's personal involvement with patients has been assumed to interfere with professional functions. Similarly, the patient's orientation toward the subjective body has been assumed to contradict the clinical orientation toward the body as an object. Thus, the concept of the professional as impersonal and objective has dictated a corresponding way of regarding the patient's body, that is, as object rather than person.

A paradigm of the sharp contradiction within the patient's experience of her body is the gynecological examination, in which a strictly impersonal definition is in force. For the patient, the part of the body being examined is often an extremely personal part of the self, perhaps the most private and emotionally invested part of the body. In the clinical situation, "the pelvic area is like any other part of the body," i.e., the individual examining the patient is "working on a technical object and not a person."[15] Any deviation from the technical attitude, e.g., by a patient's embarrassment, is countered with a repertoire of professional nonchalance, concentration on the procedure itself, and assurances that the situation is quite routine, and thus not intimate.

In the gynecological examination, the patient experiences an abrupt contradiction between her body as her own individual reality, rich with private emotional associations, and her body as sheer object, which others examine as impersonally as a technician inspects a machine. That conflict, in less dramatic form, is fundamental throughout health care, and because it can be uniquely addressed in nursing, it is important to analyze its elements and development.

The distinction between lived body and object body was indirectly indicated earlier in the discussion of the opposite perspectives of patient and professional toward the body of the patient. The distinction there was described in terms of uniqueness versus typification. That formulation expresses one aspect of the opposition, which can now be elaborated more fully.

The object body is the simpler of the two concepts for health professionals to appreciate. It is the body which the anatomist and physiologist describe, an object fully accessible upon examination and fully comprehensible by its examiner. It belongs, as do all objects, to the dimensions of quantified space and time, and to the realm of the general, the category. It is an object with parts having only functional value, not emotional, esthetic, or spiritual value: in the object body, the stomach has greater value than the hands of the concert pianist or the eyes of the painter.

The lived body is existentially opposed to the object body, but it *is not its opposite*. The lived body is not the silence of the object body when functioning well, so that one is unconscious of its objective existence as long as nothing in it breaks down. That unawareness of the body is not the lived body; it is simply a negative contingency, an experience conditional upon one's not encountering the body-as-object. As a positive condition categorically independent of and experientially prior to consciousness of the body-as-object, the lived body is not a thing at all (not even a well-running, non-intrusive thing), such as we usually denote by the word "body." Thus, it cannot be the opposite of the object body. Instead, it is a mode of orientation: the immediate, prereflective consciousness of the self *as capable of affecting its world*, as well as the consciousness of being vulnerable to the world's impact.[16]

The lived body, unlike the object body, is not in objective space and time. On the contrary, it forms its own space through its actions, drawing the world's space toward it, so to speak, centripetally.[17] Nearness and distance are a function of relevance, not measure. In the same way the lived body shapes its own time, with retension and protension interwoven and overlapping according to one's purposes, unconstrained by linearity.

It might be supposed that the lived body could be described, at least metaphorically, as an experience of interiority, but this fails for two reasons. In the first place, empirically, when the distinction between inner and outer emerges—for example, in early childhood and in illness—it is often the interior of the body which is felt to be "other," a baffling region not recognized as part of the self in the way that familiar, external features and functions are.[18] Secondly, and more important, the lived body is the self in which inner and outer *are not distinguished:* "Being-for-itself must be wholly body and it must be wholly consciousness; it cannot be *united* with a body."[19] The metaphor of interiority connotes subjectivity, privacy, privileged access—features that imply hiddenness and assume another, external, part of the self which is exposed. The lived body is thus reduced to a version, or rather, an inversion of the object body, its mirror image, when it is in fact another order of being from that of the object body.

If we understand the concepts of lived and object body as existentially opposed, and yet not logical opposites, then it is possible to recognize that the destruction of one does not automatically invoke the presence of the other (as in "if not a, then b"). It is especially important for the purposes of this chapter to recognize the transition that occurs from lived body to object body. The immediacy of the lived body is only partly mediated by illness, injury, or pain. With the appearance of incapacity, one experiences the body as something which opposes his purposes, a weighted mass, a thing-like other. Incapacity shatters the lived body. But the transition is not yet complete. The object body does not replace the lived body through illness alone. The otherness of the body in illness is rendered complete only through the category— the most essential instrument of clinical science. The category transforms "pain here" into precise, pathological phenomena which, even if one is a clinician, have no experiential relation to "pain here." The clinical view presents the patient with a body that is not his or her own, a disease process of which the patient has no direct perception. But, the new reality is objectively discernible for *others*. "Others have informed me of it, others can diagnose it; it is present for others even though I am not conscious of it."[20]

This then is the discrepancy between lived and object body, generated for the patient, first by the experience of incapacity and, second, by the perspective of science. What unique possibility exists in nursing for reconciling the opposition and restoring to the patient the unity of self and body which is prerequisite for true self-determination?

History suggests that nursing has focused exclusively upon the lived body and the object body in turn, moving from its earlier concern for immediate comfort of the patient, to the modern concern of science for the objective condition of the patient. Nursing can now surpass both of these extremes: the nurse, as advocate of the patient's wholeness, is committed to advocacy of neither the shattered lived body nor the inevitable object body. In short, nursing can make possible for the patient an enrichment of the lived body by the object body, and an enlivening of the object body by the lived body. The nurse can assist the patient to recover the objectified body at a new level at which it is neither mute immediacy nor pure otherness, but an otherness-made-one's-own, a lived objectness.

The experience of incapacity brings an awareness of the body as a being in its own right, with an irreducible reality of its own, an integrity that, so to speak, will not be compromised. The denial of that essential fact of human existence is bought at a great price: the lost possibility for enriching the self through the integration of that otherness.

It is this integration, the conscious unifying of self and body, which advocacy nursing assists the individual to achieve. The nurse assists the individual, as patient, to live the body's objectness as his or her own, instead of allowing it to remain alien. That unity is more fully expressive of one's totality than even the lived body is. The new unity is a reflective, more complex and articulated reality, inasmuch as one is now able to establish a conscious identification with aspects of his being which were previously undifferentiated, but have, through illness and objectivity, made themselves known. It is now important and possible to make them one's own, to an extent that was not important at the level of the object body, and not possible at the level of the lived body. "What threatens to estrange itself in us communicates to us *all the more* . . .that it is actually our own."[21]

It is that reconciliation of the person with the body-as-other, at a new level of integration and articulation, which nursing advocates. Nursing is uniquely able to mediate the lived/object body duality, inasmuch as it addresses both aspects of the person as one. It affirms the value of the lived body through the intimacy of physical care and comforting. At the same time, it affirms the reality of the object body by interpreting to patients their experience in terms of an objective framework—usually science, in Western cultures—which enables them to relate an otherwise hopelessly unique and solitary experience to a wider, general understanding. By continuously interrelating the two dimensions, the nurse demonstrates for the patient that the lived/object body relation is not an either/or relation, but a dialectic in which neither aspect is meaningful without the other. Both are essential, and mutually reciprocal.

This is easiest to realize when persons adhere exclusively to one or the other extreme. The modern example is the patient whose entire reality is the object body, who regards and refers to the body only in clinical terms—X-ray findings, laboratory studies, biopsy report, and so on. The more common example, given the traditional refusal to allow patients such access to their object bodies, is the patient whose only reality is the lived body, and who categorically renounces the object body as alien to the self by designating the health professional as the executor of this unwanted estate.

The challenge to advocacy nursing is to enable the individual to reclaim the aspect that has been excluded. Without incorporation of the object body, the lived body is an existentially weightless "I," unmediated and unenriched by detail, function, and form. Without the "I" of the lived body, the object body is an inanimate machine belonging to no one and everyone. Thus, the ideal of nursing is to enable patients to achieve a reconciliation, a reintegration, of these equally one-sided dimensions, in a synthesis that will necessarily be unique for each individual, and without which the self-unity required for patients' authentic self-determination will be impossible.

ADVOCACY AND THE RIGHT TO MEANING

The preceding sections have described existential advocacy in three ways:

1. the nurse's assistance to individuals in exercising their right of self-determination, through decisions which express the full and unique complexity of their values
2. a mode of involvement with patients which necessarily engages the entire self of the nurse
3. assistance to patients in unifying the experience of the lived body and the object body at a level that incorporates and transcends both

In conclusion, we can summarize advocacy nursing as the participation with the patient in determining the *personal meaning* which the experience of illness, suffering, or dying is to have for that individual.

At no time is the existential concern about the meaning of one's life more urgent than when the nature or continuation of one's existence is in jeopardy. At that point, the crucial question which the individual must answer is not "how can I secure my existence?" but "what does this jeopardy mean?" Only from the answer to that question can decisions then be reached concerning modes of treatment, forms of coping, the degree of autonomy desired, and so on. Ultimately, self-determination means the individual's own decision about the meaning of an experience, before decisions are reached about responding practically to the experience. For that meaning to be freely determined, it cannot of course be imposed by the "nature" of the person's condition, by clinical concepts of illness, or by professional notions of "loss," "disability," and "suffering." Thus, for example, the patient with terminal prostatic carcinoma is free to decide whether he shall think of his experience in moralistic terms (punishment for promiscuity), scientific terms (simply cellular phenomena), cultural terms (permission to grieve), naturalistic terms (the inevitable pain and dying that come to all), or purely individual terms which violate all of these—perhaps an inconsolable despair over the absurdity of the experience, or a decision that suffering can be a means of finding one's own way, by confronting the absurdities of existence not as defects but as necessary antitheses in the dialectical relation between joy and sorrow in human life.

For the same reason that the question of meaning arises, namely, the threat to existence, individuals require assistance in order to determine the meaning of their experience. That assistance is provided ideally by the person who has the most comprehensive understanding of the experience and who is as fully involved as the patient. That person is the nurse. The approach of nursing encompasses both care and cure, intimate concern for the lived body and scientific treatment of the object body. Moreover, the nurse offers a necessary alternative perspective which complements and completes the partial perspective of the patient, inasmuch as the focus and intensity of the nurse is directed toward the other rather than the self, and the orientation of the nurse is toward the typical rather than the solitary. Finally, the continuity with which only nursing attends the patient enables the nurse to experience individuals as unique human beings continuously engaged in creating their own histories.

No other health profession at present combines all these elements. More important, none even proposes as its ideal this reconciliation of the most radical dichotomies in health care—the unique and the general, personal intensity and professional objectivity, the body as "I" and the body as other. Nursing, by aiming at the solution of these conflicts and the human fragmentation they produce, in order that patient and nurse can participate as unified selves in the patient's process of self-determination, expresses the ideal of existential advocacy. On this basis, the nurse is the ideal professional to particiate with the patient in the decision about that which is most crucial in all experiences of illness: the meaning of the experience for the individual.

NOTES

1. Sam Schulman, "Basic Functional Roles in Nursing: Mother Surrogate and Healer," in *Patients, Physicians, and Illness*, E. Jaco (ed.), Glencoe, Illinois: The Free Press, 1958, pp. 528-537.

2. Joyce Travelbee, *Interpersonal Aspects of Nursing*, Philadelphia: F.A. Davis, Co., 1966, p. 49.

3. For elaboration of this position, see Dworkin's discussion of Mill in Gerald Dworkin, "Paternalism," *The Monist*, 56, January 1972, pp. 64-84.

4. Bernard Gert and Charles M. Culver, "Paternalistic Behavior," *Philosophy and Public Affairs*, Vol. 6, No. 1, Fall 1976, pp. 45-57.

5. This in fact is exactly what Gert and Culver argue in regard to a physician's insisting that a patient talk about an impending trauma against her expressed wishes.

6. Paternalism thus attributes to the person affected a form of ethical egoism, i.e., the belief that individuals (patients, in this case) *ought* to act in such a way as to promote their own good, with the altruistic footnote that if they fail to do so, action will be initiated on their behalf to obtain the good for them until such time as they resume the moral duties of egoism.

7. Sandra Kosik, "Patient Advocacy or Fighting the System," *American Journal of Nursing*, April 1972, pp. 694-698.

8. The goals of patient advocacy programs may not even be solely those of consumer protection. Improving patient compliance and smoothing over patient complaints are often hidden or explicit objectives. (*Ibid.*, 209) Even when the primary goal is helping patients, advocacy can function as a defense for

professional decisions: "patients experiencing a token economy wanted to know whether the therapy team was violating patients' rights... All it took here was an explanation that token economy is a medically approved, widely accepted mode of treatment. The patients were more accepting of it after that." Wanda Nations, "Nurse-Lawyer is Patient-Advocate," *American Journal of Nursing,* June 1973, pp. 1039-1041.

9. Professor Engelhardt's concern here that "paternalism in the interests of health" is being replaced by a "paternalism in the interests of authenticity" is, fortunately, unfounded. I am proposing advocacy as an ideal, not as a duty, norm, prescription, or imperative which conceivably might involve "enforcement." Moreover, it is simply contradictory to believe that we can force persons to act in an unforced way. The ideal of assisting patients to exercise their freedom does not entail that they be stigmatized for declining, just as the ideal of health presumably does not entail that patients be punished for disdaining modern medicine. Authenticity, like health, is ultimately fashioned and confirmed only by the individuals themselves; professionals can assist the process but they cannot command it.

10. Friedrick Nietzsche, *The Anti-Christ* (R. J. Hollingdale, trans.), Baltimore, Penguin Books, 1969, p. 118. See also Nietzsche, "The will to suffer and those who feel pity," *The Gay Science,* (Water Kaufman, trans.), New York: Random House, 1974, pp. 269-271.

11. Max Scheler, *The Nature of Sympathy* (Peter Heath, trans.), Hamdon, CT.: Archon Books, 1970, p. 9. (emphasis added).

12. *Ibid.,* p. 15.

13. *Ibid.,* p. 46.

14. Another example of resolving the personal/professional dichotomy, this time through physical involvement between nurse and patient, can be developed around the importance of touch in nursing. For a discussion of the laying-on of hands in nursing care, see Dolores Krieger, "Therapeutic Touch: The Imprimatur of Nursing," *American Journal of Nursing,* May 1975, pp. 784-787.

15. Joan P. Emerson, "Behavior in Private Places: Sustaining Definitions of Reality in Gynecological Examinations," in *Readings on Ethical and Social Issues in Biomedicine,* Richard W. Wertz, (ed.), Englewood Cliffs, New Jersey: Prentice-Hall, Inc., 1973, pp. 221-233.

16. I am grateful to J. Melvin Woody for his insistance upon the vulnerability of the lived body, elaborated in "Helping the Patient Survive: Some Remarks on Prof. Sally Gadow's essay 'Existential Advocacy: Philosophical Foundation of Nursing'" (unpublished).

17. Sartre captures this phenomenon of lived space in his analysis of "the look," in which the world is experienced, not as fixed in uniform space, but "perpetually flowing" toward me, its center. See *Being and Nothingness: An Essay in Phenomenological Ontology*, (Hazel Barnes, trans.), New York: The Citadel Press, 1969, 232ff.

18. This is contrary to Sartre's account of the distinction, in which the object body emerges as the exterior part of my self which the other perceives, "extended outside in a dimension of flight which escapes me. My body's depth of being is for me this perpetual 'outside' of my most intimate 'inside'" (Sartre, *op. cit.*, p. 328).

19. *Ibid.*, p. 281.

20. Herbert Plügge, "Man and His Body," in *The Philosophy of the Body: Rejections of Cartesian Dualism*, Stuart F. Spicker, (ed.), New York: Quadrangle/The New York Times Book Co., 1970, p. 305.

21. *Sartre, op. cit.*, 332.

5

The Nurse-Patient Relation: Some Rights and Duties

Dan W. Brock

My concern in this chapter is to elaborate a view of the moral situation of the modern nurse, and of some of the rights and duties that define the moral context in which she works. I shall be looking at some of the moral claims that she possesses and some of the moral constraints on her, as well as the moral claims and constraints of others that impinge on her. I shall attempt to bring out some of the respects in which her unique situation raises moral issues not found in, or at least not prominent in, other areas of biomedical ethics. It would, however, be a mistake to think that all or even most of the serious moral problems she faces are not instances of problems that arise in other areas of biomedical ethics, just as most of the moral problems of biomedical ethics are instances of moral problems arising in other areas of social and political life.

NORMATIVE VIEWS

Since many persons concerned with moral issues in nursing are not professional philosophers, it may be helpful to review very briefly some ways in which the principal normative, ethical theories, or positions diverge. The kind of moral position or view one appeals to in a discussion such as this will influence not only the positions or "solu-tions" proposed for particular moral conflicts and problems, but will affect as well which problems are identified as moral problems, and the way in which those problems are characterized or conceived.

This brief review of different normative views and how they differ should also suggest some of the points where we can expect to find disagreement on specific moral issues in the area of nursing, as well as some of the more basic sources of this disagreement. Finally, the sort of moral view one holds is likely to affect the account one offers of the nurse-patient relationship, as well as, perhaps, the nurse's other rela-tionships within the health-care team.

One common moral view is that which Ronald Dworkin has called goal-based, and which is more commonly termed consequentialist, utilitarian, or teleological.[1] Most generally, it views morality as con-cerned with the production of desirable or valuable experiences, com-monly human happiness, desire satisfaction, welfare or well-being.[2] How one ought to act morally in any situation is determined by how possible alternative actions tend to promote or frustrate these goals, and the right action is that action which, among alternatives open to a person, maximizes these valuable consequences for all persons affected.

The consequences for any one person count no more than those for any other person. It is a matter of the amount of human happiness or welfare produced, not of who gets it. The morally significant features of persons in the goal-based view are ultimately their roles as the sub-jects or recipients of the experiences the theory holds to be valuable. Any assertions of moral rights or duties are justifiable, if and only if, recognizing them will in the case at hand promote the maximization of human happiness or welfare. And this means, I believe, that the dis-cussion of moral issues in such a consequentialist, moral view could dispense with talk of moral rights and duties entirely, to be replaced with an account of the consequences of various actions for human well-being.[3] If we think reference to moral rights or duties is indis-pensable for at least some moral problems, then we shall have to reject the consequentialist moral view.

The two other moral theories or positions that I shall mention here are what philosophers commonly call deontological. Each one makes an appeal, at the most basic level, to a different sort of moral notion with a logical form carrying implications for the sort of actions that are morally justified, as well as for the general focus the view employs. These are what Dworkin has labeled duty-based and rights-based moral views. Both provide, though in different ways, for the moral evaluation of human action based not solely on the consequences of that action for the production of valuable experiences. Both hold that at least some actions that violate moral rights or duties are morally wrong even if they maximally promote valuable experiences or goals; they hold some sacrifice of valuable goals to be justified in order to protect moral rights or to conform to moral duties. No plausible moral theory will entirely ignore the extent to which actions produce valuable experiences, and so the strength of duties or rights in an overall moral view can be measured by the amount of valuable experience that can be justifiably sacrificed in order to meet our duties and respect people's rights. A duty-based moral view can be seen as positing a moral ideal for a person in the form of a set of moral commitments, constraints, or prohibitions of behavior that can be violated only at the cost of one's moral integrity, at the cost of becoming morally evil or corrupt. Such prohibitions will usually concern what one deliberately does to other persons, what are sometimes loosely called one's projects, as opposed to, for example, what one simply fails to prevent. The basic moral categories of a duty-based view are all constraints or limits on our action to which we must conform. These constraints commonly derive from a general conception of relations between persons, and the moral requirement that what we do to other persons be justified by features of that person, and our relation to him.[4] Duty-based views attempt to account for the intuition that a person has a special responsibility for what one deliberately and directly does to others; this is different from one's responsibility for, and for affecting, the actions of others. In this sense, duty-based views take more seriously the distinction between persons than do goal-based views, and focus on persons as agents whose own deliberate actions put them into morally significant relations with specific other persons.

Finally, compare a view whose basic moral principles ascribe moral rights to persons. Rights function differently from duties in that they delineate areas in which the person possessing the right is at liberty to act as he or she sees fit, i.e., to act in one's own interest, as opposed to delineating specific constraints to which one must conform. Rights specify, as well, areas of behavior in which it is wrong, at least without special justification, for others to interfere with the rightholder's exercise of the right, or to fail to provide that to which the rightholder has a right, if and when he or she calls for it. They thus create claims or entitlements against others. We may choose to exercise our rights or not, waive them, and so forth, as we see fit. Rights-based views emphasize a view of persons as capable of forming purposes, of making plans, of weighing alternatives according to how well they fulfill those plans and purposes, and of acting on the basis of this deliberation. Rights protect our ability to exercise these capacities, capacities whose exercise is often associated with the idea of autonomy, independent of how doing so promotes production of the valuable experiences the consequentialist focuses on. Moral rights delineate and protect areas in which we are to be left free to decide what direction our life will take, even in cases where others may with good reason disagree about whether our decision is for the best; they are especially suited to providing a person with control over specified areas of his or her life.

We might then summarize that in a goal-based view, morality is concerned with the production of valuable experiences; in a duty-based view, with the conformance of human action to prohibitions necessary to the maintenance of relations between persons and moral integrity; and in a rights-based view, with the exercise and preservation of moral rights and the free choice they protect.

Two possible confusions should be removed at the outset. First, I shall speak of both rights and duties or obligations of the nurse and others. Moreover, philosophers commonly point out that rights and duties are correlative, i.e., if Jones has a right, for example, to be told the truth, at least some other Smith has a duty to tell him the truth, and vice versa.[5] How then are rights-based and duty-based views to be distinguished if rights always come with duties, and duties always come with rights? The important point is that it matters whether it is rights or duties which are appealed to as basic or ultimate moral principles—those principles beyond which no further appeal is possible in the justification process, and, in turn, whether it is rights and duties that are only derivative. First, it matters because of the general nature or structure of the moral view, the general "picture" of morality and the person it embodies. And it has one other implication important for our purposes here—if rights are basic, then in general the duties derivative from them can be cancelled or wiped out if the right is waived by the right-holder, e.g., the right not to be killed possessed by a terminally ill patient. However, if duties are basic they need not be cancellable in this way, that is, on the voluntary request of the person against whom the duty holds. If, for example, a duty never to take innocent human life is morally basic, then such a request from a terminally ill patient is a request that one act evilly, and is to be resisted.

The second point that needs clarification is the relation between the distinctions that I have employed concerning different moral views and the moral views actually held by real persons. Few of us fall neatly and completely into one of these three moral camps, but rather most persons feel at least some of the plausibility of each of these three ways of looking at moral issues. This can take two different forms which are worth distinguishing. First, on a single issue a person may be attracted to conflicting moral positions on that issue. He or she experiences what might be called *intra*personal conflict on the issue. Second, a person may find that different areas of moral experience may require different sorts of moral principles (i.e., goals, duties, or rights) as basic to be able to account for one's moral views there. This means that the complete moral view consists of a specific, often quite complex, combination of the three sorts of moral principles or conceptions as delineated above.

Finally, I want to suggest in the most general and brief terms how one's account of the nurse's rights and obligations is likely to differ according to the underlying moral theory appealed to. First, on a goal-based moral theory that takes the promotion of, let us say, human happiness or welfare as basic, how the nurse ought to act morally in the various circumstances in which she finds herself will be determined in each instance by a calculation of how possible alternative actions will promote the welfare of all affected. The nurse's professional duties ought to be defined in a manner that maximally promotes human welfare, and exceptions to such duties will be morally justified whenever making exceptions best promotes human welfare. Likewise, any rights that the nurse and more especially the patient have stop at the point where recognizing them in any particular case would fail to maximize human welfare. To take an example, a nurse has no moral duty not to deceive a patient or to obtain his or her consent for treatment, nor has the patient any moral right not to be deceived or to have his or her consent obtained, if deception or treatment without consent will in the case at hand maximally promote the welfare of all affected. Nor should the patient's welfare have any precedence in the nurse's calculations, except to the extent that the patient's welfare is likely to be more affected quantitatively than will that of other persons. In the goal-based view then, everything will depend on the expected consequences for human welfare of alternative actions, and moral disagreement will be reduced to empirical questions about expected consequences.

If moral duties are taken as basic, while some others such as the physician and patient will have duties towards the nurse, the emphasis in any such account of her moral context will likely be on the various moral duties that constrain her behavior towards others. The nurse's professional duties to provide various forms of care and services, which ought to be derived from more basic moral duties, will together form a picture of how a *nurse* ought to act, and her general moral duties not to deceive, kill, and so forth, will form a picture of what a moral *person* must do. Any moral rights that others, and especially the patient, have against the nurse, must be derived from her more basic duties. Such a moral view will consist largely of an elaboration of a set of constraints and requirements on her, constraints and requirements that cannot be justifiably breached merely because doing so in a particular case will best promote human welfare.

On the other hand, if moral rights are taken as basic, the nurse will have rights that others must respect, while the moral rights most fully and significantly determinative of the situation are likely to be those of the patient. It is the patient's mind and body that are being acted on in various ways. It is the patient who is especially vulnerable to various sorts of harms that would violate his or her rights. Moreover, as I will elaborate below, it is the patient's rights that are necessary to explain central elements of the nurse-patient relationship. If we begin with the patient's rights, then we should expect that there will be significant aspects in which the nurse's moral context will be determined by the way in which the patient exercises those rights.

NURSE-PATIENT RELATIONSHIP

I want to turn now to a brief consideration of the nurse-patient relationship. In so doing I shall appeal primarily to what I call a rights-based moral view. I do so because, in general, I consider such a view to be most acceptable, and because, in particular, moral rights seem to be essential to an adequate account of the relation of the nurse and the patient. There are at least two sorts of moral considerations relevant to a full understanding of the moral relationship between the nurse and the patient. First, there are general moral considerations, rights and duties, that the nurse and patient would have simply as individuals, apart from their roles as nurse or patient (e.g., on most any moral theory it is prima facie wrong to kill or seriously injure another human being, and this holds for persons generally, not merely for nurses and patients). Second, there are moral considerations that arise only out of the particular relationship that exists between a nurse and patient, just as there are in other relationships such as parent and child, public official and citizen, and so forth. A complete account of the nurse's moral situation must include both sorts of considerations, and would be far too complex and lengthy to attempt here.

I shall emphasize considerations of the second sort, and even then my discussion will not be at all comprehensive. On virtually any account of the nurse-patient relationship, the nurse owes at least some care to the patient and the patient has a right to expect that care. However, this is not an obligation that the nurse has to just anyone, but only to the patient, nor a right a person has toward just anyone, or even toward any nurse, but rather only toward his or her nurse. How then do nurse and patient get into this relationship at all? IF we pose the question in this way, I think it is clear that the common alternative accounts of the nurse-patient relationship cannot all be plausibly construed as even possible answers to this question, and that more generally, they address two different questions—some speak to the origin of the relationship, how it comes about, while others speak to the nature or content of the relationship. I think a clearer understanding of the relationship is gained if we separate these two issues, because the account of the origin of the relationship will affect in turn the account of its content. Consider six of the more common accounts of the relationship of the role of the nurse vis-à-vis the patient:[6]

1. The nurse as parent surrogate
2. The nurse as physician surrogate
3. The nurse as healer
4. The nurse as patient advocate or protector
5. The nurse as health educator
6. The nurse as contracted clinician

I do not want to deny that nurses do not at times, and at times justifiably so, fill each of the first five of these roles. And at least most of these first five roles refer to professional duties a nurse assumes in entering the profession of nursing. But how is it that a nurse has any duty to perform in any of these roles toward a particular person (patient), and how is it that a person (patient) has any right to expect a particular nurse to perform in these roles? Only the last model, the nurse as contracted clinician, can explain that. We must be able to make reference to a contract, or better an agreement, between the two to explain these roles. This point may be obscured somewhat by the fact that what a nurse would do for a patient in any of the first five roles can be generally assumed to be beneficial for the patient, or at least intended to be beneficial. If it is for the patient's good, why must the patient agree before the nurse is permitted to act? But just imagine someone coming up to you on the street and giving you an injection, even one intended to be, and in fact, beneficial to you. A natural response would be, "You have no right to do that," and underlying that response would likely be some belief that each person has a moral right to determine what is done to his or her body, however difficult it may be to determine the precise nature, scope, and strength of that right. Or, imagine a strange person in a white uniform coming up to you and lecturing you about the health hazards of your smoking or lack of exercise. Well-intentioned though it might be, a natural response again might be, "What business is it of yours, what right do you have to lecture me about my health habits?" Again, the point would be that it is a person's right to act in ways detrimental to his health if he chooses to do so and bears the consequences of doing so. This particular right usually derives from some more general and basic right to privacy, liberty, or self-determination (autonomy). Yet both these actions are, of course, of the sort frequently performed by nurses toward their patients. Likewise, any duties of a nurse to provide care to a particular person cannot derive simply from the duties she assumes in the nurse's role, nor can the right of a particular patient to nursing care from a specific nurse.

If we think of the nurse-patient relationship as arising from a contract or agreement between the nurse and her patient, then these otherwise problematic rights and duties become readily explicable. The patient contracts to have specified care provided by the nurse, in return for payment by the patient, and the patient in so doing grants permission to the nurse to perform actions (injections, tests, and the like) that she would otherwise have no right or duty to do. In agreeing to perform these duties, the nurse incurs an obligation to the patient to do so, as well as a right to be paid for doing so.

A natural objection to such an account is that it appears to rest on a fiction, since in the great majority of cases nurses and patients never in fact make any such agreement; rather, the patient finds himself in a physician's office, or in a hospital, where the nurse as a matter of course performs certain tasks, while the nurse, if she makes any such agreements at all, makes them with the physician or the hospital that employs her. This reflects the fact that the provision of health care is considerably more complex and institutionalized than any simple nurse-patient account would suggest, but it does not, in my view, show the contract or agreement model to be mistaken. The patient makes the agreement generally with the physician or the hospital's representative, and that agreement is to have a complex of services performed by a variety of health-care professionals. The nurse is an indirect party to this agreement, and can become committed to it, by having contracted or agreed with the employing physician or hospital to perform a particular role in the health-care process.

A related objection to this account is that at these intervening agreement points, it is still often the case that the contract or agreement never takes place, certainly not to the extent that what is to be done is spelled out in any detail, and so the account still rests on a fiction. But these agreements can and do have implicit terms, terms which can be just as binding on the parties as if they had been explicitly spelled out. These implicit terms are to be found primarily in the generally known and accepted understanding of the nature of such health-care relationships, and in the warranted social expectations the involved parties have concerning who will do what in such relationships. The content of such expectations will in large part derive from the nature of the training of various health-care professionals, the professional codes and legal requirements governing their conduct, as well as more general public understandings of their roles.

Why insist on a contract or agreement model of the nurse-patient relationship that requires an appeal to agreements between intervening parties, as well as to implicit terms that are generally not spelled out? The reason is that such an account makes one fundamental point very clear. That is, that the right to determine what is done to and for the patient, and to control, within broad limits, the course of the patient's treatment and care, originates and generally remains with the patient. One important reason for insisting on this is that it is insufficiently appreciated and respected by health-care professionals. Many health-care professionals hold that if they reasonably believe that what they are doing is in the best interests of the patient, that is sufficient justification for doing it. However, in my view, this is a serious mistake because it does not take an adequate account of the patient's right to control the course of treatment.

An important part of at least one common understanding of the physician-patient relationship, and in turn of the patient's other health-care professional relationships (including, but not limited to, the nurse), is that the health-care professional will, with limited exceptions (e.g. public health problems arising from highly contagious diseases), act to promote the best interests of his or her patient. Treatment recommendations and decisions are to be made solely according to how they affect the interests of the patient, and ought not be influenced by the interests or convenience of others.[7] The patient's confidence that the health professional will act in this way is especially important because of the extreme vulnerability and apprehension the ill patient often feels, the patient's inability to provide his or her own necessary health care, and the patient's often very limited capacity to evaluate for himself whether a proposed course of treatment and care is in fact for the best. This focus on the patient's interests to the exclusion of others, however, is different from, and should not be confused with, physicians' or nurses' being justified in acting in whichever manner they reasonably believe to be in the patient's best interest.

The right of the physician or nurse to act in the patient's interest is *created* and *limited* by the permission or consent (from the patient-nurse/physician agreement) that the patient has given. To take two extremes, a patient might say to the physician or nurse, "I want you to do whatever you think best, and don't bother me with the details," or the patient might insist on being fully informed about all factors and alternatives concerning the treatment and on retaining the right to reject any aspect of that treatment. In my view, should the patient desire it, either of these arrangements can be justifiable, as well as, of course, many modified versions of them. This has the important implication that the various expectations concerning what the health professional will do, which generally give content to the nurse-patient relationship, only partially determine that relationship. It is also subject to modification that is determined principally by what the patient desires of the relationship, and how he or she in turn constructs it. This is the other difficulty, besides their failure to explain how the relationship comes into being between particular persons, of the five alternatives mentioned above to the contract or agreement model of the nurse-patient relation. One cannot speak generally about the extent to which the nurse ought to act or has a duty to act, for example, as health educator or parent surrogate, because it ought to be the patient's right to determine in large part the extent to which the nurse is to take those roles. What the patient wants will often become clear only in the course of treatment, but to put the point in obligation language, the nurse's obligation is in large part to accommodate herself to the patient's desires in these matters.

I have been considering only the case of patients who satisfy conditions of competence, that is, persons who possess the minimal cognitive and other capacities necessary for forming purposes and making plans, weighing alternative courses of action according to how they fulfill those purposes and plans, and acting on the basis of this deliberative process; such persons are able to form and act on a conception of their own good.[8] Some of the more difficult moral problems in health care generally arise in cases where these conditions of competence are not satisfied, e.g., with infants and young children, with persons suffering from extreme senility or some forms of mental illness.[9] However, I think that we must first understand the nurse-patient relation in the case of the competent patient, before attempting to determine how that relationship may have to be modified when the patient is not competent. It may, then, be useful to consider what the contract or agreement model of the nurse-patient relation, with its emphasis on the patient's rights, might imply for some typical moral problems the nurse encounters with the competent patient. Common to many such problems insofar as they involve only the nurse and her patient (later in the chapter I shall take up some complications that arise from her relationship to other health professionals) is a conflict between what the patient wants and believes is best, and what the nurse believes is in his best interests, in the interests of all persons affected, or morally acceptable. Consider the following cases:

Case 1. Patient A has requested his nurse to inform him fully of the nature of his condition and of the course of treatment prescribed for it. However, the treatment called for, and which the nurse believes will be most effective in his case, is such that given her knowledge of the patient, she believes that fully informing the patient will reduce his ability and willingness to cooperate in the treatment and so will significantly reduce the likely effectiveness of the treatment. What should she tell him?

Case 2. Patient B instructs his nurse that if his condition deteriorates beyond a specified point, he considers life no longer worth living and wishes all further life-sustaining treatment withdrawn. The nurse believes that life still has value even in such a deteriorated state, that it would be wrong for the patient deliberately to bring about his own death in this way, and, in turn, wrong for her to aid him in doing so. Should she follow his instructions?

Case 3. Patient C, after being fully informed of principal alternative treatments for his condition, has insisted on a course of treatment that the nurse has good reason to believe is effective in a substantially smaller proportion of cases than an alternative treatment procedure would be. She considers the additional risk in the rejected treatment, which seems to have affected the patient's choice, completely insignificant. Should she insist on the more effective treatment, for example, even by surreptitiously substituting it, if she is able to do so?

Each of these cases lacks sufficient detail to allow a full discussion of it, and in particular, each artificially ignores the presence and role of other health-care practitioners, most notably the physician, who is generally prominent if not paramount in such decision making. I shall bring the physician into the picture shortly, but the cases are instructive even in this oversimplified form. Case 3 is perhaps the least difficult. It would be permissible for any interested party, and a duty of the nurse according to her roles as health educator and healer, to discuss the treatment decision with her patient, and to attempt to convince him that he has made a serious mistake in his choice of treatments. But just as the patient should be free to refuse any treatment for his condition if he is competent and so decides, he is likewise entitled to select and have the treatment that the nurse (or physician, for that matter) would not choose if it were her choice; the point simply is that it is not her treatment and so not her choice. She has no moral (or professional) right to insist on a treatment the patient does not want, even if it is clearly the "best" treatment, and it would be still more seriously wrong to surreptitiously and deceptively substitute the treatment she prefers.

Case 2 can be somewhat more difficult because it may at least involve action in conflict with the nurse's moral views rather than a conflict over what course of action is, all things considered, medically advisable, as in Case 3. Case 2, of course, raises the controversial issue of euthanasia and the so-called right to die. This is a complex question that I have considered elsewhere, and here I only want to note that Case 2 involves only fully voluntary euthanasia, generally accepted to be the least morally controversial form of euthanasia.[10] I shall suppose here that a patient's right to control his treatment, and to refuse treatment he does not want, can include the right to order withdrawal of treatment even when that will have the known and intended consequence of terminating his life. If we interpret the nurse's view that life under the circumstances in question would still be worth living as merely her own view about what she would do in similar circumstances, then her view is relevant only to what she would do if she were the patient and nothing more; it entails nothing about what should be done where it is another's life and his attitude to it that is in question. She would not waive her right not to be killed in these circumstances, but the patient would and does, and it is his life and so his right that is in question. I would suggest as well that a mere difference over what it is best to do in the circumstances (apart from moral considerations) does not morally justify the nurse's refusal to honor the patient's expressed wishes. However, her difference with the patient may be a moral one, in particular she may hold as a basic moral principle that she has an inviolable moral duty not to kill deliberately an innocent human being. In that case, to assist in the withdrawal of treatment in order to bring about the patient's death will be according to her moral view a serious wrong, a serious evil. The nurse's professional obligations to provide care should not, in my view, be understood to require her to do such, just as she should not be required to assist in abortions if she believes that fetuses are protected by a duty not to take deliberately an innocent human life. While there should be no requirement in general for her to participate in medical procedures that violate important moral principles that she holds, that of course in no way implies that another nurse who does not hold such duty-based views about killing should not assist in the withdrawal of treatment. (Of course, if she holds killing to be wrong because it violates a person's right not to be killed, then she will correctly reason that the patient in Case 2 has waived that right, and so no conflict between her moral views and what the patient wants will arise.)

Finally, consider Case 1. The "Patient Bill of Rights" proposed by the American Hospital Association specifically allows that "when it is not medically advisable to give...information to the patient" concerning his diagnosis, treatment, and prognosis, such information need only "be made available to an appropriate person in his behalf" but need not be given to the patient himself. This would seem clearly to permit the nurse to withhold the information from the patient in Case 1. However, I believe the Patient's Bill of Rights is mistaken on this point. This is a particular instance of a general overemphasis on and consequent overenlargement of the area in which health professionals should be permitted to act towards patients on the basis of their own judgment of the "medical advisability" of their action toward the patient. It is perhaps natural that health professionals, who are trained to provide medical care for patients and who undertake professional responsibilities to do so, should consider medical advisability a sufficient condition generally for acting contrary to a patient's wishes, and here for withholding relevant information from the patient. But once again, as long as we are dealing with patients who satisfy minimal conditions of competence to make decisions about their treatment, unless the patient has explicitly granted the nurse the right to withhold information he seeks when she considers it medically advisable to do so, medical advisability is not sufficient justification for doing so. Our moral right to control what is done to our body, and our right, in turn, not to be denied relevant available information for decisions about the exercise of that right, do not end at the point where others decide, even with good reason, that it is medically advisable for us not to be free to exercise that right. In general, one element of the moral respect owed competent adults is to respect, in the sense of honor, their right to make decisions of this sort even when their doing so may not be deemed medically advisable by others, and even when those others are health professionals generally in a better position to make an informed decision. When other health professionals are in a better position to make an informed decision, a patient may have good reason to transfer his rights to decide to them, or to allow himself to be strongly influenced by what they think best, but he is not required to do so, and so they have no such rights to decide for him what his treatment will be when he has not done so.

I want to emphasize that, in my view, moral rights generally, and in particular the rights of the patient relevant in the three cases above, are not absolute in the sense that they can never justifiably be overridden by competing moral considerations. But such justifiable overriding requires a special justification, and that human welfare generally, or the welfare of the person whose right is at issue, will be better promoted by violation of the right is *not* such a special justification.[11] Thus, rights need not be absolute in order to have an important place in moral reasoning. Cases involving young children and noncompetent adults are important instances where specifically paternalistic interference with a person's exercise of his rights can be justified.

Perhaps the point of emphasizing the contract or agreement between the patient and the health care professional is now a bit clearer. That contract model emphasizes the basis for and way in which the right to control the direction one's care will take ought to rest with the patient. It is not, of course, that the nurse is mistaken in taking her role to be a healer, or health educator, for these are important professional services she performs, but rather that her performance in these roles ought to be significantly constrained and circumscribed by the rights of her patients to control what is done to them and their bodies.

NURSE-PHYSICIAN/HOSPITAL RELATION

Until now, my discussion of the nurse's situation has focused on her relations with her patient, and this narrowed focus has made the discussion unrealistic in at least one important respect. Specificially, the fact that the nurse generally operates in a hierarchic, institutional setting in which she is in the employ of others—hospitals, physicians, and the like—has been ignored. Many of the moral uncertainties and conflicts that nurses experience concerning their duties and responsibilities derive from their role in this hierarchical structure, and from questions about their consequent authority to decide and act in particular matters. The patient has a place in such issues, but the issues do not arise when only the nurse and patient are considered. Now I want to fill in the picture some by considering briefly this nurse-physician/ hospital relation. It might seem tempting to maintain that since the physician's and hospital's relation to the patient ought to be understood in terms of the same agreement or contract model as the nurses, it ought to be possible to talk generally of the patient-health-care professional relationship. Differences in specific duties and rights of nurses as opposed to other health-care professionals would derive only from the division of labor and differentiation of function within the health-care setting. Since all health-care professionals ought equally to be constrained by the rights of the patient, and since all ought to advise, decide, and act on the basis of the interests and rights of the patient, there should be no conflict among health-care professionals in general, and among nurses and other health-care professionals in particular. There is, in principle, an important truth in this point, but I doubt that any nurse would recognize this as an accurate or realistic account, however oversimplified, of her situation, and so we must see where it goes wrong. The basic point is an obvious one. Conflicts arise because the nurse has conflicting roles, as agent for the patient but also as employee of the hospital or physician. These roles can conflict in at least two significantly different sorts of ways. First, the nurse can find herself in disagreement with other health-care professionals, in whose employ she is, over what is in fact best for the patient. Second, physicians, hospital administrators, and the like, as well as the nurse herself, have other roles and in turn other interests besides that of acting to serve the patient's health needs, and these interests can come into conflict with the patient's interests.

The potential for conflicts of both sorts for the nurse is probably increased by the relatively low degree of autonomy nurses currently possess in comparison with many other professionals. One aspect of the notion of a profession and professional is the assumption that there is a body of knowledge the professional has mastered, which others generally do not possess; this has contributed to the idea that professionals ought to be able to decide jointly with their clients how they will practice their profession with a high degree of autonomy and freedom from control and regulation by others outside the profession. Nurses, however, generally work for a hospital or physician, and so are largely under the direction and authority of that employer. This is unlike many other professionals like architects, lawyers, and physicians, who are either self-employed, or in the employ of the client whose interests are to be served. I suspect that this fact about the current status of nursing—a profession with an increasingly large body of technical knowledge that has been mastered, but with quite limited autonomy in acting on that professional knowledge without control and direction from others—contributes importantly to the uncertainty about its role and status to which nursing as a profession seems to be subject.

With this said, it is also worth noting the extent to which many of the conflicts that nurses face are endemic to participation in social activities generally, and are only accentuated by the nurse's limited professional autonomy and the complexity and role differentiation that characterizes modern medical care. Whenever persons combine together in a cooperative activity that requires some common group decision to be made about how the activity will proceed, possibilities will arise for our personal, moral, or technical judgment concerning what ought to be done to conflict with the group decision, however this latter is arrived at. The point can be made clearer by distinguishing two sorts of conflicts that arise in moral life, and for that matter in nonmoral questions, concerning which action is preferable among alternatives. In one sense, any interesting and perplexing moral problem involves conflict between competing moral considerations, whether they be rights, duties, consequences, or whatever. If one can find no significant reason whatever, for example, to deceive another person, then it will be generally conceded that it would be wrong to do so, and most of us would experience little if any uncertainty about the question. Case 1 was more difficult just because the deception seemed necessary for the beneficial treatment consequences. The nurse in deciding what to do must confront this conflict, and in coming to a decision about what all things considered she ought to do, she weighs these conflicting considerations against each other in order to decide which is more important or overriding. But in the simplified circumstances of Case 1, once she decided what all things considered would be right, she can proceed to do that. When the activity becomes more complex, with many different persons with different training, knowledge, and moral views, cooperating in some joint enterprise, as is the case in most modern medical care, a new sort of conflict commonly develops. The treatment team must now decide as a group how to proceed and whether, for example, the patient can be justifiably deceived by the withholding of information when doing so seems medically advisable. No matter what the group decision process, only if the nurse had sole and final authority to decide could she be guaranteed that the group decision would not be one she considered mistaken or wrong. And of course, if anyone involved in medical care has such sole, decision-making authority, it is physicians and not nurses. Even if nurses gain an increased role in decision making, they are not likely to attain a dominant role in the foreseeable future, and so will continue to face this problem of whether to act in the manner the group, or the physician, has selected, even when they believe that such action will be not in the patient's best interests, or will be morally wrong. There are then conflicts of judgment, both medical and moral, that arise from the group nature of medical care, and conflicts of professional role that arise from possibly conflicting duties to the patient, hospital, physician, and the nurse's own family, among others. Other things equal, we should attempt to arrange social life so as to minimize particularly deep conflicts of this sort, but they are not going to be soon eliminated.

What can be said about how these conflicts ought to be resolved, and how the nurse ought to proceed when faced with them? These are conflicts generated by the nurse's professional duties and roles. In general, the important point is that her professional duties and responsibilities ought to be defined and interpreted so as to maximally respect and protect the patient's right to control the course of treatment. It is this moral right of the patient that is ultimately the principal justification of any professional duties the nurse has, for example to follow within some limits the physician's judgment regarding the indicated treatment; such professional duties should be understood to be dependent on and derived from the patient's prior moral rights. And that means, in turn, that such a professional duty can be overriden when following the physician's judgment is clearly contrary to the best interests and express desires of the patient. This primacy of the patient's moral rights over the nurse's professional duties and responsibilities to others like the physician is of fundamental importance, but it fails to bring out the full complexity of the decisions nurses face in such role conflicts. The range of considerations relevant to such decisions can be considerable, even within a generally accepted framework that assigns primacy to the patient's rights. I strongly doubt that any simple and comprehensive principles could be developed that would provide satisfactory guidance concerning how these considerations should be weighed over a wide range of concrete cases. All that can usefully be attempted here is to take one such case and illustrate what some of the relevant considerations would be in the nurse's attempt to reach a judgment about how to respond in the situation.

Consider a case similar to Case 1 above where a nurse is explicitly instructed by the attending physician to withhold certain information from the patient concerning his condition on the grounds that he believes it would be medically detrimental to the course of treatment for the patient to be fully informed. Suppose now that the patient asks the nurse for the withheld information. What kinds of considerations are relevant to the nurse's decision about what to do?

1. Is this physician's decision within accepted medical, and hospital, practice in this case? Is the nurse's following the physician's directive in cases of this sort required by accepted standards of professional nursing practice?

Only if the answer to one or both of these questions is negative will she be able to protest (e.g., to others in the hospital or medical hierarchy) about this particular order of the physician as opposed to general medical practice in such cases, or to be within her professional rights in acting contrary to his directive. If the answer is affirmative to both questions, then the nurse will have a professional duty to withhold the information as directed, though that will not fully settle the moral question.

2. Who ought to make decisions of this sort concerning withholding of information from patients?

The nurse may or may not believe that the existing decision-making process for such questions should be changed, quite apart from her views about what the content of the decisions made should be. Nurses commonly, and in my view rightly, argue that their role in health-care decision making should be increased from what it now is, and so this may be an area where appropriate action includes protest of and attempts to change the way such decisions are made;how such protest would most effectively be made, and to whom, depends on the context. However, change of the decision-making process is likely to be a long-term matter and so not helpful to her with the case at hand. Alternatively, she may not believe the decision-making process requires change at all, despite her disagreement with this particular decision.

3. What alternative courses of action are open to the nurse in the case at hand if she remains convinced the physician's directive is wrong, despite its accordance with existing medical practice?

Relevant alternatives include: discussing the issue with the physician in an attempt to get him to change his decision; protesting this decision to others in the medical hierarchy; acting on the physician's order while trying to change the decision process; acting contrary to the physician's directive with the likely personal loss involved, such as disciplinary action or loss of job; attempting to withdraw from the case; resigning her position, perhaps coupled with protests concerning the physician's action to others (e.g., the hospital and media). Which of these alternatives, or combinations of them, is the most advisable will depend on a variety of considerations such as the likelihood of her protest being effective, the personal cost to her in making it, the likely effect of her withdrawal from the case on what is done to the patient, and so forth.

Notice that none of the above depends directly on the issue being about withholding of information—these are considerations and alternatives that arise independently of what the specific conflict in roles concerns. However, the seriousness of the harm done to the patient by the action she has been ordered to perform will, of course, also be relevant to the nurse's overall decision. For example, if what had been ordered was "not to resuscitate," without the knowledge and against the will of the patient, a more serious wrong to the patient would be in prospect than in the case at hand, and a more serious obligation would fall on the nurse to attempt to prevent that wrong.

This very brief sketch of some morally relevant considerations in the decision about what to do in role conflicts and conflicts of duty that nurses face, does not take us very far towards resolutions of such conflicts. However, I believe no general, authoritative principles or pronouncements indicating how such conflicts should be resolved would be both helpful and defensible. Instead, once we recognize the pervasiveness of such role conflicts in nursing practice, the next step must be the detailed consideration of the concrete instances of these role conflicts in their full complexity and diversity.

NOTES

1. Ronald Dworkin, *Taking Rights Seriously*, Ch. 6 (Cambridge, 1977). My characterization of the three types of moral views owes much to Dworkin's discussion. I have employed a discussion very similar to that in this chapter for somewhat different purposes in my "Moral Rights and Permissible Killing," in *Ethical Issues Relating to Life and Death*, (ed.) John Ladd, New York: Oxford University Press, 1979. The general distinction between teleological and deontological theories is discussed in almost any ethics textbook;see, for example, Richard Brandt, *Ethical Theory*, Englewood Cliffs: Prentice-Hall, 1959, William Frankena, *Ethics* 2nd Ed., Englewood Cliffs: Prentice-Hall, 1973, or Paul Taylor, *Principles of Ethics*, Encino, Calif.: Dickenson Publishing Co., 1975.

2. It makes some difference which of these notions is used to formulate the utilitarian position, though I shall not pursue the matter here. I have discussed this, as well as other issues in the formulation and assessment of utilitarianism in my "Recent Work in Utilitarianism," *American Philosophical Quarterly*, 10, 1973, pp. 241-276.

3. It is because of the nonessential role of moral rights and duties in consequentialist views that the approach to social policy questions commonly called cost/benefit reasoning is properly understood as a form of consequentialism.

4. A very suggestive discussion of the moral constraints that derive from the idea of relations between persons, with specific application to problems in war, can be found in Thomas Nagel, "War and Massacre," *Philosophy and Public Affairs*, 1, 1972, pp. 123-144.

5. This is discussed in many places, for example, Brandt, *op. cit*. Ch. 17, and, with specific reference to the political context, Stanley Benn and Richard Peters, *The Principles of Political Thought*, Glencoe, Ill.: Free Press, 1964, Ch. 4. In fact, I believe the inference from rights to duties is considerably more plausible than the inference from duties to rights.

6. I have drawn these from the very helpful paper by Sally Gadow, "Humanistic Issues at the Interface of Nursing and the Community." See *Connecticut Medicine*, Vol. 41, No. 6, June, 1977, pp. 357-361.

7. Such a view, with specific reference to the dying patient, is advocated in, among other places, Leon Kass, "Death as an Event: A Commentary on Robert Morrison," *Science*, 173, August 20, 1971, pp. 698-702. To what extent this account of the physician-patient relationship is defensible, or is in fact adhered to in practice by physicians, is problematic.

8. Plans of life, and their relation to a conception of one's good, are discussed in John Rawls' *A Theory of Justice*, Cambridge, Mass.: Harvard University Press, 1971, Ch. 7; and Charles Fried's *An Anatomy of Values*, Cambridge, Mass.: Harvard University Press, 1970.

9. For philosophical accounts of the principles of paternalism relevant to treatment of the incompetent, see, for example, Gerald Dworkin, "Paternalism" in *Morality and the Law*, (ed.) R. Wasserstrom, Belmont, Calif.: Wadsworth Publishing Co., 1971; and John Hodson, "The Principle of Paternalism," *American Philosophical Quarterly*, 14, 1977, pp. 61-69. I have discussed paternalism with specific reference to the mentally ill in "Involuntary Civil Commitment: The Moral Issues," in *Mental Illness: Law and Public Policy*, (eds.) Baruch Brody and H. Tristram Engelhardt, Jr., Dordrecht, Holland/Boston, Mass.: D. Reidel Publishing Co., 1980.

10. I have discussed some implications of a rights-based view for euthanasia in my "Moral Rights and Permissible Killing," *op cit*. See. also the paper by Michael Tooley, "The Termination of Life: Some Moral Issues," in the same volume.

11. For one attempt to specify the general limits of such special justifications, see Dworkin, *op. cit.*, Ch. 7.

6

The Nurse's Role in an Interest-Based View of Patients' Rights

Bertram Bandman and Elsie Bandman

INTRODUCTION

We hear from a number of quarters that there ought to be a moratorium on "rights" talk. So it is a pleasure to find an essay such as Dan Brock's that provides an elegant and engaging defense of moral rights in the nurse-patient relation.

The view of rights presented there identifies rights with freedom, and with such important values as respect for the patient's autonomy and dignity. This account of rights is undoubtedly steeped in a laudable and venerable tradition. But is this the only view of rights? Does a view of rights which identifies rights with freedom of choice provide an adequate account of the role of rights?

We will want to consider this view of rights not only to endorse its real and important strengths but also to assess what difficulties or inadequacies, if any, there might be within it. If there are some objections, we may wish to consider an alternative view of rights which takes into account rights of another kind.

The contention of this chapter is that there are some difficulties in the freedom-based view of rights and that an alternative view of rights provides a more helpful account of moral rights in the nurse-patient relation.

NURSE'S ROLE IN A FREEDOM-
BASED VIEW OF RIGHTS

After identifying three moral positions, adapted from Ronald Dworkin, goal-based or utilitarian, duty-based, and rights-based, Dan Brock defends the third of these positions, one that is generally favorable to a rights-based view. He reveals the difference it makes to a nurse in her or his relation to patients to hold a view oriented primarily by one or another of these views. He says that rights provide "a person with control over specified areas of his life and "Rights protect our exercise of . . . capacities . . . whose exercise is often associated with autonomy." He views a patient whose rights are respected and honored as one who is regarded as free to make up his or her own mind, one against whom deception, lies, and manipulation constitute a gross moral violation.

Brock then applies his rights-based view to three cases. The first, Case A, involves a nurse who has the problem of deciding whether to withhold information or tell what she knows to the patient, an event which will set the patient back. The second, Case B, concerns a conflict between a seriously ill patient who requests treatment withdrawn if deterioration continues and a nurse who considers it wrong to assist in a patient's death. The issue in the third case, somewhat like the first, is whether the nurse should, if necessary, deceive the patient about the course of treatment. All three cases involve a conflict between paternalistic intervention and a patient's right to decide on the basis of fully relevant information.

In each case a patient's right to decide takes precedence over that of the health team including the nurse. This means that the patient makes the choice, which is very much like an example Stanley Benn cites of having a right to drink oneself to death, even though it is not in one's best interest to do so.[1] The single principle of one's right to decide what happens in and to one's own body seems to cover all three cases equally.

There is, however, one overstatement, namely, the right "to control what happens in and to one's body," which seems to be an odd right. Can we actually control what happens in and to our bodies? The notion of a right as a form of control might be appealing if it were possible and therefore practical to speak of rights in this way. But it does not seem to be so when there are things that no one can do anything about to control what happens in and to his body. This sort of notion of what a right can do reminds us of Alf Ross's notion of rights as "tu tu's," a form of verbal magic, things no one can seriously believe in.[2]

If one had a right to control what happens in and to one's body, someone else or some group would presumably have the corresponding duty to protect and provide for this right. For if one really has rights, presumably others, such as health professionals would have corresponding duties. As Kant noted in a similar connection, to have a right is to have "the capacity to obligate others."[3] But who could be the recipient of such a duty? Health professionals, nurses, physicians? Could they possibly carry out all that would be required to control what happens in and to one's body? There is no technology to effectively purify all sorts of substances in the very air we breathe. To impose such a duty on anyone or everyone to control what happens in and to people's bodies would be a sheer technical impossibility. Furthermore, there do seem to be restrictions even on a person's right to his or her body. A person with a contagious disease ought to have rights in and to his or her body limited, for example.

However, Brock's point that to have rights means that a nurse's role in the performance of her duties "ought to be significantly constrained and circumscribed by the rights of her patients" to have their choice taken seriously concerning "what happens in and to their bodies" is an important contribution to the concept of rights; and the analysis of this right may give us a reason for postponing a moratorium on "rights" talk. This kind of right and the venerable theory that has been invoked in its defense has recently been called "the will" or "choice" theory of rights,[4] one that we will want to consider later on in these remarks.

128   BANDMAN AND BANDMAN

SOME OMISSIONS AND DIFFICULTIES

One puzzling omission is that despite the adroit application of goal, duty, and rights-based moral views to the nurse-patient relation, we note no reason given for the absence of a reference to one of the mainsprings of ethics for most nurses, notably the Agapeistic or Love ethic espoused, for example, by St. Paul and St. Francis. It is, for example, not entirely clear why a nurse should not also be influenced by a love-based moral position.

One could also make a defensible case favoring a duty-bound and even a goal-based moral position. One need not be a consequentialist to recognize that there are things no inconsequentialist can afford to ignore. Even justice, it has been held, is justified by the good it brings. Rights are similarly useful; otherwise considering their strengths and weaknesses is pointless.

There is another difficulty. The position has been taken that the nurse should not have to comply with a patient's rights if her moral view is different from the patient's, as in "assisting in abortion." There is a seemingly easy way out. Another nurse will come along and not be similarly constrained.

If a patient's rights imply corresponding duties on others, including nurses, what happens if a nurse with a conflicting moral view is the only one around or if all the available nurses oppose the patient's view? What happens to the patient's right to "constrain and circumscribe" the nurse's treatment?

Let us imagine the following: Nurse N. and patient B. are the only survivors of a small, commercial plane crash in a remote area of Alaska. B. is suffering third-degree burns and is trapped under the right fuselage and appeals to N. to assist in his or her death. N. knows that there is no help nearby and no hope of lifting the fuselage or of treating B., whose condition is hopeless. Yet N. is morally opposed to killing.

If the rights of the nurse and not those of the patient are uppermost, then the patient is effectively stripped of whatever rights he or she might really have had, in this case to terminate life. A right is not a right if it can be denied because a nurse's moral view does not, as it happens, coincide with a patient's rights in the matter. One has to decide who has rights in such matters.

Anti-Paternalism

The heart of the matter, however, seems to be an underlying assumption favoring a form of anti-Paternalism that seems at times more stout-hearted than a defensible form of anti-Paternalism needs to be, even on behalf of the centrality of patients' rights which has been put forward.

The right to control one's body and one's treatment and the emphasis given to self-determination, privacy, freedom, autonomy, the "express desire" of the patient, the emphasis on not being deceived, and being given complete and truthful information, all point to an important aspect of a rights-based view, namely the role of an individual patient's will in individual decision making.

Undoubtedly, a cornerstone of rights is the plank of freedom noted by Hart[5] and Rawls[6] and before them by Mill[7] and Kant.[8] Freedom is undoubtedly a vital condition for having any right.[9] There is also little doubt that anti-Paternalism in health care on behalf of abused patients' rights is a welcome relief from the repeated undermining of individual patients' rights. But we want to explore the assumption of those who hold great store and faith in the will.

The tradition of anti-Paternalism assumes the importance of the "will," revealed at times by the emphasis given to subordinating the "patient's best interest" or "the patient's good" or what is "medically advisable" to the "patient's desire" or to "the express desires of the patient."

The defense of a patient's exercise of his or her own will is revealed in such important ideals as privacy, liberty, and self-determination. We wonder whether faith in the sovereignty of the will can be strongly justified.

In forwarding a form of anti-Paternalism, one assumption even explicitly held in Brock's discussion of the three cases is that the patients involved are all "competent."

Do the sick not rather slide in and out of "competence?" In developing a criterion of competence, Joel Feinberg suggests that we distinguish direct from indirect forms of killing. By overeating, smoking, and driving unsafely we engage in indirect killing. But, Feinberg says, by slashing our wrists or chopping off our hands with an axe we engage in direct killing which marks our behavior as incompetent.[10] It seems easier to identify clear cases of incompetence, but the fuzzy borders under the heading of "indirect killing" do not make it altogether obvious that a person's judgment is not impaired.

Gerald Dworkin cites Mill's stout defense of anti-Paternalism, in defense of one's liberty and against unjustified interference. According to Dworkin, to Mill "the burden of proof is always on those who propose" to restrain another person's freedom.[11] As Dworkin eloquently puts it, according to the defense of liberty presumption, "better ten men ruin themselves than that one man be unjustly deprived of liberty."[12]

To Mill the only grounds for interfering with another's freedom are "self-protection" and "harm to others."[13] In Mill's distinction between self-regarding and other-regarding actions, the burden of proof is on the state's coercive apparatus to show that it is entitled to interfere with a person's self-regarding actions. To prevent harm being done to others, appropriate interferences with a person's other-regarding actions are justified.

But the presumption of libertarians, following Mill, is that they should have sovereignty over self-regarding actions, which include one's right "to control what happens in and to one's body," and "to control one's treatment." This right includes also the right to decide when and if to withhold life-saving treatment, even if that leads to one's death. As long as they are competent, patients have a right to decide.

Yet Mill finds exception to not interfering with a person's liberty involving self-regarding actions. Mill's emphasis on identifying a person's right with an enlightened rather than an "uninformed or misinformed choice," in Feinberg's terms, is brought out in Mill's bridge example as follows:

If either a public officer or anyone else saw a person attempting to cross a bridge which had been ascertained to be unsafe and there were no time to warn him of his danger, they might seize him and turn him back, without any real infringement on his liberty; for liberty consists in doing what one desires, and he does not desire to fall into the river.[14]

Mill had another exception besides a person unknowingly doing something which that "person does not desire," namely that a person may "not sell himself into slavery."[15] We might compare limitation on freedom in selling oneself into slavery to consigning oneself to death. If Mill's principle justifies paternalistic interference in the case of slavery, it would seem to justify paternalistic interference even more strongly to prevent a person from unknowingly seeking his or her own death or harm, as the case of the bridge illustrates.

There are then limits to one's control, self-determination, liberty, privacy, and autonomy not provided for by some anti-Paternalists. As an officer may stop a person from walking on an unsafe bridge, what about a medical officer stopping a patient from doing analogous things to his or her body by not following what is "medically advisable" and what is in one's interests in health matters? Are these always to be subordinated to expressions of freedom of will, even in cases where one's own liberty would be augmented by imposing rational restraints on it?

Patients may not know what is best, and even when medically advised, may do things to their bodies that are harmful. It seems that an excessive form of anti-Paternalism does not compromise the liberty of patients, no matter how ill-advised such a course may be.

There seems to be some connection, however, between a patient's capacity for judgment and knowing what is best, such that if one acts too often by disregarding what is known, one's place on the competence scale slides off into incompetence. The relation between a patient's will and judgment and knowing what is best is insufficiently shown by this sort of excessive anti-Paternalism. If we have less and less reason to believe in the assumption that the patient knows best, what are we to say of a patient's competence to decide how to keep from falling off the bridge and how to keep from (what that person would consider to be a case of) harming his or her own vital interests?

It does not seem that one's vital, rational interests, especially if they enhance one's liberty, must in some cases necessarily be subordinated to one's express desires and expressions of will, especially those of the moment. Identifying one's rights with one's will and desire rather than one's vital, rational interests is not the only way to decipher one's real rights as a patient. If the patient's expressed desires are the major or even complete indications of a patient's rights, then there may be somewhat too few limits on a patient's liberty. (Counseling and advising, imploring, and even coaxing and berating by nurses and others are sometimes not enough to get patients to do what would be rationally the best course for them.)

However, there are limits, justifiable limits, it seems, on a patient's liberty, privacy, self-determination, and capacity to control what happens in and to his or her body and limits also to control the course of our treatment. There are grounds of justified interference with one's liberty both for one's own interests as well as for the good of others. One may have to be restrained from taking heroin, from otherwise unknowingly harming himself by taking medically inadvisable forms of treatment, or by failing to prolong his life where the evidence may well warrant doing so in terms of the viability of one's life.

Regarding justified interferences with one's liberty for the good of others, one is restrained from spitting on the streets or speeding on the highways; one is required to take a blood test prior to marriage, to have vaccinations, be restrained from poisoning the water supply, or spreading contagious diseases.

Virtues such as freedom and autonomy are precious but they may not be the only virtues associated with having rights. Furthermore, freedom, too, has limits in the form of rational constraints on what a person may do in and to his or her own body as well as what a person may do to others. And the reasons for these constraints may give us some reason to doubt that one's competence to judge is solely implied by expressions of will. There is something to be said for connecting one's rights also to at least knowing often enough what is in one's interests. If the patient doesn't quite often enough know best, how competent can such a patient be? What is the relation between a patient's knowledge, his or her competence, and his or her freedom to decide what to do in and to his or her body?

If the concept of competence is connected to the assumption that the patient knows best, an assumption we have increasing reason to doubt, according to Hart, no less,[16] we may then have correspondingly increasing reason to have less confidence in staking as much as we once did on the underdefined concept of competence. If the patient too frequently does not know what is best for what is in his or her own interest and for what is in the interest of others, there may be reason to question the lack of limits of anti-Paternalism, and in particular, to question the connection between a patient's rights and a patient's freedom.

We nevertheless do not wish to conclude this portion of our remarks without endorsing the relation of rights to freedom. For, as has been argued convincingly elsewhere, there are no rights without freedom. It is only that there also cannot be freedom without limits, limits that augment freedom, and accordingly no rights without limitations on freedom, limits and strictures not clearly enough present in the attempt to assimilate rights to freedom exclusively. Anti-Paternalism, yes, but not without restrictions in accordance with justified classes of exceptions.

CRITIQUE OF THE "WILL" THEORY OF RIGHTS: AN ALTERNATIVE VIEW

Although Brock has given us one view of rights, there is an alternative rights-based view that takes into account rights of another kind.

Adopting a distinction made earlier by H.L.A. Hart, D.N. MacCormick distinguishes between a will-based theory of rights, which emphasizes virtues associated with freedom, and rights of another kind, an interest-based theory, which emphasizes benefits conferred equally on all persons regardless of their capacity to exercise their wills. These benefit rights include the right of children to "care and nurture," for example, and are associated with rights of assistance.[17]

A will-based theory stresses such treasured rights as the right to "informed consent." A will-based view of rights confers on each individual a space, a territory, zone or domain where he or she is sovereign. This tradition places great weight on one's body. One reads and hears over and over that if there are any rights at all, they are rights in and to one's body. The will-based view of rights is a champion of privacy and freedom.

An interest-based theory of rights stresses the need for food, shelter, clothing, health care, education, and other basic conditions of subsistence necessary to live.

A look at the United Nations *Universal Declaration of Human Rights* shows that Articles 1-21, which include the right of free speech and the right to vote, sometimes called political rights, are oriented by a will-based theory. Articles 22-27, however, which include the right to a decent standard of living for everyone, including adequate housing, shelter, medicine and health care, including maternity benefits, guaranteed employment, and periodic holidays with pay, are oriented by an interest or needs-based theory of rights. In contrast to the first kind, these are sometimes called "social and economic rights" or "rights of social justice."[18]

Some writers such as D.D. Raphael call the first kind "rights of action" and the second kind "rights of recipience." Other writers such as Martin Golding call rights of the first kind "option rights" and refer to the second kind as "welfare rights." Golding includes the rights of the comatose and the rights of infants and children under welfare rights.

One need not defend some recent excesses concerning these benefit rights, (rights which could not possibly imply corresponding duties on the parts of others), to hold, however, that an account of rights that fails to take account of those who cannot act on their own behalf, such as infants, children, the handicapped, and those others too impoverished to know their rights, does not provide an adequate account of rights. For there are rights which those who cannot act on their own behalf, including the incompetent, nevertheless have—namely, benefit or subsistence rights such as the right to (be helped to) live and the related rights not to be harmed and, if necessary, even to be helped. Rights of this kind have a crucial bearing on deciding some life-and-death issues quite differently from the answers one would give on the basis of a will-based theory of rights. Moreover, the satisfaction of these benefit or subsistence rights provides the very conditions for achieving freedom rights and the associated virtues of autonomy, dignity, and self-respect.

A rights-based view such as the one presented by Brock turns out to belong to one tradition of rights—the liberty tradition. It is an important and influential view, but it is, as some recent writers have shown, not the only tradition. There is even a question as to whether the liberty rights tradition is even the prevalent tradition, and whether rights of a second kind, namely rights to receive assistance (welfare or benefit rights) may not limit the scope of the older option or liberty rights.

The emphasis on the liberty rights tradition may also reveal a reluctance to deal with patients who are either comatose or not competent. Liberty rights do not explain what to do with infants, the unconscious, and the incompetent, except to rule them out of the pale of their being rights recipients. However, infants, the comatose, and the unconscious do have rights, as Golding has pointed out, only rights of another kind, namely welfare or benefit rights. Rights of the second kind, namely benefit rights, are rights not only to be left alone, but to receive assistance, including care and nurture; and this has also to be accounted for in any moral rights-based view.

To show how such omitted rights may affect a rights-based view in nursing, we present the following hypothetical example:

The patient AC is a woman who has had several near-fatal attacks while hospitalized. Consequently, she has developed high anxiety about her condition and lives in fear of dying. She often asks for the latest laboratory reports, and insists on knowing every last detail concerning her treatment and prognosis. A study demonstrably convinces the health team responsible for AC's treatment that high anxiety is decidedly detrimental to this particular patient in this condition, that the only way to ease AC's high anxiety, which they believe could, if unrelieved, result in the next (fatal) attack, is to tranquilize the patient. But AC, fearful of losing control, refuses all tranquilizers. The health team decides to prevent her from knowing that she is on tranquilizers. Are they wrong?

A case could be made, it seems, showing that the health team was well within the bounds of respecting the rights of this patient. A case might be made in favor of this patient's rights, it seems, even if in the above case it means withholding information and even doing something to the patient's body to which she has not even consented. In a pinch, the right to live and also the right not to be seriously harmed, on an interest-based view of rights, seems more fundamental even than the right to be free or even the right not to be deceived under the above type of circumstances.

A second hypothetical example of an admittedly difficult case is that of a patient who requests withholding of treatment if his condition deteriorates. Our suggested example is not so dramatic as Elsie Bandman's would-be suicide case whom the nurse saves from death by successfully restraining the patient on the ledge of a window.[19] However, this does seem to us to provide a counter-example of identifying respect for a patient's rights by doing whatever the patient wants, including the withholding of life-saving treatment.

Our suggested second case is of a man who feels that further deterioration makes life no longer viable. Should the nurse always comply with the patient's right to decide to live or die? Our hypothetical case goes as follows:

> The patient requests treatment withdrawn if deterioration continues. But the nurse knows other patients who felt the same way when wracked with pain, until they were administered a research drug which brought about a remission. In the case at hand, the nurse believes that a temporary shortage of this vital drug will be alleviated soon. She has persuaded the health-team members to give high priority to this patient's needs on just and equitable grounds. The nurse and other health-team members believe that if the drug arrives soon, there is hope for a remission and resulting improvement of the patient's present medical condition. The nurse thinks that the patient would consider it in his own interest to live if he could know the likelihood of the drug's arriving in the near future and the likely effects of the drug on his condition. But the team thinks it inadvisable to tell the patient of this drug until it actually arrives and he is actually among the selected recipients, which is probable but not certain. If the research medication does not arrive or if the patient is not selected, it would have been a needless cruelty to raise the patient's hopes by informing him of this possibility. They would feel responsible for the patient's death should the individual then commit su-

icide. The team members in committee meetings discuss their feelings. They do not think this is paternalistic in any sense other than one they would want in a rational contract situation were they the patient. They compare the patient's plight and their role in refusing to withhold treatment to Mill's officer forcibly preventing the man about to enter an unsafe bridge from doing so. Furthermore, this team agrees that assisting the patient to withdraw treatment is not foreclosed. Only to withhold treatment at this time, before the drug arrives, would be to agree to a possibly avoidable death were the nurse now to comply.

One could thus override a freedom-based right, expressed by a patient's "desire" and "control over his or her treatment" by considering the rights of patients in similar conditions and concluding with what any rationally interested person would want in that situation. One could override a person's will-based rights by considering a person's own more fundamental, deep, interest-based rights. Is such a nurse violating the patient's rights? Liberty rights, yes, but one's benefit rights?

NURSE'S DIFFICULTIES IN KNOWING THE PATIENT'S TRUE WISHES

The nurse in some difficult cases will need to consider the problem Elsie Bandman[20] poses in applying Michael Walzer's dilemma[21] toward deciding what Shakespeare's Brutus really wants. Brutus, we may recall, earlier in *Julius Caesar*, renounces suicide, and although married to Cato's widow, frowns on Cato's own suicide. Later, when Brutus faces the prospect of being marched in triumph as a prisoner in Rome, being vanquished and overrun, he asks three friends, one by one, to assist him in his death. After each friend refuses, Brutus, turning to a servant, finds a person willing to oblige.

If a nurse sees herself or himself, as Elsie Bandman suggests, as a friend and ally rather than as a servant or instrument to be used, her response will be different. Is our nurse who refuses to kill patient B like Clitus who says "I'll rather kill myself"? Or is our nurse like Volumnius who says "That is not an office for a friend," or like Strato, the servant, who when asked wants to make sure this is Brutus's wish by saying "Give me your hand first"? Elsie Bandman, in the essay referred to, poses the issue: Does a nurse treat the killing of a patient like a contract consummated by a handshake?

If a nurse knows that there is still a viable and enjoyable life to be lived, in which retrospectively Patient B could after a time say, "Thank you for not listening to me when I asked you to withhold treatment and to assist in killing me," then the nurse would be like Volumnius or even Clitus. Or is our nurse like Strato, the servant, willing to oblige on a handshake, taking B's request at face value? If she or he takes the servant Strato's role, the nurse becomes B's servant, not his friend, one who presumably knows and cares for B. On the option-liberty-will theory of rights, the nurse will be the servant, an instrument willing dutifully to assist the patient who is taken at his or her word as the sovereign over his or her body. On the benefit-rights-based view the nurse will be more apt to be the friend of the patient, more like Clitus, Dardanius, or Volumnius than Strato the servant; for such a nurse will act on behalf of interests which the patient would on retrospect and in a rational frame of mind want for himself or herself.

If the nurse is like Clitus, preferring death to harming or killing the patient, this may make a nurse appear paternalistic, perhaps a "mother surrogate," one who knowingly cares for the interests of her patient.

In this case, the patient may still want to die, let us suppose. But what if our nurse in the case above instead attempts to and succeeds in saving the patient's life against the patient's will of the moment? We do not think such a nurse could seriously be said to have wronged the patient. Ordinarily to deprive a person of his or her rights is to do something wrong to that person. But that can't quite be said about this type of case. For the patient could conceivably be grateful afterwards for having been saved.

To protect the real rights of a patient it may take a theory of rights but not one that takes a patient at face value as a servant might, but rather as a friend would, one who more deeply knows and cares. The kind of theory of rights this might require is not the older political liberty rights theory, the one which says, "Don't interfere," but the newer one which says, "Help me." "Assist me."

TOWARD A MORE ADEQUATE
THEORY OF RIGHTS

An adequate theory of rights, we've been suggesting, does not discount "the express desires of the patient," or the patient's will and all. For such a theory of rights would be impoverished if it did not also take account of the interests which a patient in a rational state would have wanted for himself or herself. To think of one's interests is to think also of one's retrospective self. And who knows this but a nurse acting as the patient's friend at a time of life when he or she knows that what is most needed is not a servant to obey his or her every command but one who knows the real person? A theory of rights that speaks to a patient's real needs at such a time, one that penetrates into the latent, deeper meaning of a patient's being, one that protects a patient's vital rational interests, such a theory seems the more adequate one at such a time.

Being deceived and being treated without consent are serious breaches of one's liberty rights. But there may be other rights, rights even more closely tied to one's right to life, such as the right not to be harmed and even to be helped when in need which takes priority. What if one's judgment is temporarily impaired and one refuses to consent, but afterwards would have cause to regret the decision made; do we as his or her friend not have a duty to aid in protecting his or her most fundamental rights to life, health, and happiness, even if our doing so means that the patient is temporarily deceived or that we do something of which the patient (temporarily) does not approve?

The circumstance of serious illness may compel the most stouthearted of us to the role of recipients, where our liberty rights, which are normally at the foreground in most other life circumstances, recede and are in escrow while deep rights, background rights, rights of recipience, interest-based rights, come to the foreground.

That is why we might prefer our nurse at the final invoking of our rights to be a friend rather than a servant. And we may know friends who would even deceive us to prevent harm coming to us. And if friends are like Clitus, they would rather die themselves.

No wonder, perhaps, that such rights, rights of assistance, may be regarded as supererogatory, Good Samaritan rights, rights not easily fulfilled, rights easily scoffed at and rejected, a cause of steady ridicule and derision, and abusively referred to as "frivolous," "utopian," "too expensive," "unrealistic," and "pie in the sky." Some would call these acts of love or friendship or benefit no rights at all, which if not forthcoming would entitle a person to sue. Yet these rights, sometimes termed "programmatic rights," "incipient rights," "manifesto rights," "proposed rights"—names given to such rights by various recent writers—make a powerful appeal to enlightened principles of justice. These strange looking "rights" become the forerunners of legal rights. As pressing claims to rights, they transform the way we come to think about rights.

Such rights have their counterpart when they are unmet or violated. The violation of these rights evokes the moral outrage of growingly large numbers of human beings, not moved by force of arms or bent on destruction. Instead, the upholders of such rights are aroused by the unsatisfactory consequences of patent injustices into exposing and confronting grossly unfair inequalities, previously ignored. They are the rights we would not relinquish if we could; for stripped of these, we would have no others. Among all the rights we have, these are the ones we take most seriously. They are the deep, "background rights" that justify interferences with our freedom for the sake of the equal and greater freedom and also well-being of ourselves and others. For such rights are most closely associated with social and economic justice, which provides the conditions for the subsequent exercise and enjoyment of political freedom rights. These deeper rights are also identified with a choiceless Paternalism and love that is sometimes associated and understood by some nurses as "care." One writer, Joel Feinberg, regards these rights as "mandatory rights," which because they rule out choice, paradoxically for him are the death blow of rights; and yet he too acknowledges that they are the seed and source of all other rights, ones for which he expresses sympathetic identification.

Perhaps the source of our perplexity about such rights dates back to our puzzlement about the scope, power, and limits of the older natural rights, rights which are now expressed as the newer human rights. Or perhaps these rights consist merely in banal, freshly detected inequalities, which if so does seem to justify a moratorium. The argument of this chapter is that this is not the case, that the multiplication of rights is caused by the revelation of injustices, including those caused by the excesses of freedom-based rights.

INTEREST-BASED THEORY OF RIGHTS

Whatever the intricacies of the debate between Hart and MacCormick and others on the distinction between these two kinds of rights—freedom rights and benefit rights—defended respectively by the will theory and the interest theory, we want to suggest another way to view the cases presented. That is, to consider that the patients have not only liberty rights but benefit rights. To have rights to health and medical benefits means that to be helped medically is their right and therefore the basis of physicians' and nurses' duties. The rights of patients A, B, and C are not just rights to be left alone and to have their wills and desires respected. These rights include the right to be helped to recover and to be as effectively treated as possible. It is in that more total sense, taking into account not just his or her will and desire but all of his or her interests, that the patient is to be regarded as sovereign or alternatively in Martin Buber's language as "holy."

While will-based rights like the right to give "informed consent" and the right not to be deceived and manipulated come under the heading of freedom rights, admittedly discussed by some anti-Paternalists, interest-based rights like the right to (be helped to) live and the right not to be harmed (and even to be given some assistance) may well come under the heading of benefit rights.

Whatever such benefit rights include, which at the hands of some writers may indeed be excessive in the way of conferred benefits, that there are such moral rights, it seems, is of concern and relevance to our three cases. For appeal to such benefit rights may reveal how judgments respecting and honoring the rights of patients may well (although not necessarily) go the other way from the way an advocate of freedom-based rights would have it. Specifically, the patients in these cases who need help need the freedom to decide, but they need something in addition; they need help in the form of health benefits, which are their most fundamental rights as patients, the rights to have their lives protected and helped when they are helpless. These patients' rights, in turn, imply the duties of nurses and health professionals.

Some anti-Paternalists identify a patient's rights with his or her sovereignty of will in all three cases. But one could, we suggest, defend patients' rights by identifying rights rather with the benefits to be conferred by respecting their rights to live and to be free of avoidable harm even to the extent of overriding their own freedom-based rights, including even the right not to be deceived under special circumstances, which may constitute justified (temporary) interferences with a patient's *prima facie* sovereignty.

The protection of rights is too important to be left to individual right holders at times when they (actually) slide in and out of competence and do things they would later regret, had they acted without interference (even though they may officially be designated as "competent"). As with the officer on Mill's unsafe bridge, the members of the health team including the nurse normally have, it seems, a duty to turn back such a patient. For a patient's "liberty" consists in doing what he or she "desires" and a patient desires to live without harm.

The right to be free is treated by Mill as an immunity right in the sense that one is not free to sell oneself into slavery. To have an immunity right of this kind means one cannot (at least very easily) waive instances of the right nor relinquish the right itself.[22] This right which prevents one from selling oneself into slavery blocks legislatures from passing laws that could otherwise legalize slavery. One cannot divest oneself of the right to be free in the sense of relinquishing the right.

The right to be free importantly includes the right not to be deceived, and if the right not to be deceived can also be regarded as an immunity right, this means that one (again) cannot (easily) *waive* instances of the right nor *relinquish* the right itself.

The right to live may similarly be regarded as an immunity right, and this also means one cannot (easily) *waive* instances of it, nor *relinquish* the right itself. Indeed, of the two rights, if both were regarded as immunity rights, it would normally seem more difficult to justify waiving the right to live than to justify waiving the right to be free or the right not to be deceived.

We doubt, for example, that a patient who identified with his or her freedom and with not being deceived would say to a nurse, "You may deceive me." But the same patient, one who cares for freedom and for not being deceived, may retrospectively say to a nurse, "I can forgive you for having deceived me in this instance. After all, my life hung in the balance. It was probably the only way." One could retrospectively *waive* instances of one's right not to be deceived for the sake of fulfilling one's desires and interests by specifying, for example, that it was to save life or avoid harm.

We do not wish to champion lying and deceit and vacate the patient's freedom-based rights, but there are circumstances where a rational person could conceivably waive instances of the right not to be deceived while not relinquishing the right itself.[23] Prisoners of war are known to surrender their freedom. They thus waive instances of the right without relinquishing the right to freedom itself. For although imprisoned, they try to escape. So it is possible to waive a right to be free but only by appealing to a deeper, more fundamental right, one that "trumps" and overrides a competing right.[24] Such a right is the right to live and with minimal harm. One only waives instances of a right to be free or not to be deceived temporarily under a set of exceptions that any rational person would consider justified, if not prospectively then retrospectively, and only for the sake of a right to live or to avoid harm. The right to live, however, cannot be waived without the irrevocable relinquishing of that to which the right refers; it is thus a last stop right.

Even if, as some lawyers contend, immunity rights cannot by definition be waived, they can, by some special provision, one that coincides with our intuition in such matters, be regarded like the right of the man on Mill's bridge; if not set aside, they can be held in *escrow* or *blinked at* during an agreed class of justified exceptions. Thus, every person in serious illness will not be informed (and even misinformed) if what is otherwise known by that person will directly and demonstrably (seriously) harm or kill that person. If one doubts this justification, one might consider the following hypothetical possibility: What if we came upon a race of people who if they knew the truth would be led to instant panic and suicide? Would we not have reason to reconsider the doctrine of informed consent as well as will-based rights?

One might finally object that not everyone at all times desires to live and that the right to life, the most precious right, is one that can ultimately be waived, and that one might desire to waive one's right to live. For it is possible that the right to life under extremely painful and mutilating circumstances, fraught with hopelessness and fear, does make one's life no longer worth living, like the man on Mill's bridge who wishes to fall off the bridge. If we were the nurse who is a friend to such a patient, after considering with the patient that this is the most serious right there is, the least waivable (since for each person it can be waived only once), and if that patient's interests indicated that death was appropriate, we might then help, as the nurse should in the case of the burning plane where there is no alternative to a painful death. And if, as with Brutus, there is no friend who would help, then that will be the time for the patient to look for the assistance of a servant. Perhaps some such intuition is reason enough for holding that even the right to live is not absolute or finally unwaivable. Only the right to live without harm seems, of all rights, to be the most entrenched and most restricted from being (lightly) waived.

We have only suggested here that immunity from being (too easily) waived provides us with a way of recognizing some rights as more fundamental than others, that even on a rights-based view there are differences between rights, rights which make life and not doing harm more valuable rights than even not deceiving patients, when deception becomes necessary to save their lives or not do harm to them.[25]

CONCLUSION

The main objection we have then to some anti-Paternalist accounts of rights is that they present a will-based view of rights as if it were the whole of a rights-based view, when there is also an interest-based view of rights which both complements and may, in crucial cases, even point to a more fundamentally important kind of right than a freedom-based right.

As D.N. MacCormick says:

Freedom of choice is a good, but it is not necessarily the only good.[26]

The right to live and to do so with minimal harm and ill health may also be a good and in a pinch the defense of these other rights may sometimes matter even more than having a choice.

NOTES

1. S. Benn, "Rights," in P. Edwards (ed.), *The Encyclopedia of Philosophy*, Vol. 7, New York: Macmillan, 1966, p. 197.

2. A. Ross, "Tu Tu's," in Lord Loyd of Hampstead (ed.), *Introduction to Jurisprudence*, London: Stevens, 1972, p. 556.

3. I. Kant, "There is only one innate Right," in E. Kent (ed.), *Law and Philosophy*, New York: Appleton Century Crofts, 1971, p. 121.

4. H.L.A. Hart, "Bentham on Legal Rights," in A.W.B. Simpson (ed.), *Jurisprudence*, Clarendon, Oxford University Press, 1973, pp. 171-201.

The term "theory" in our chapter refers to the attempt to provide some sort of defensible account. This use of "theory" is found in moral, political, and legal philosophy and is not analogous to the use of the term "theory" in the physical and (possibly some) social sciences.

5. H.L.A. Hart, "Are there Any Natural Rights?" in A. Melden (ed.), *Human Rights*, Belmont, California: Wadsworth, 1970, pp. 61-74.

6. J. Rawls, *A Theory of Justice*, Cambridge: Harvard University Press, 1971, p. 302.

7. J. Mill, *On Liberty*, London: Everyman Library, 1948.

8. I. Kant, "There is only one innate Right."

9. See B. Bandman, "Some Legal, Moral and Intellectual Rights of Children," in *Educational Theory*, 27, No. 3, Summer, 1977.

10. J. Feinberg, *Social Philosophy*, Englewood Cliffs, N.J.: Prentice Hall, 1973, pp. 46-49.

11. G. Dworkin, "Paternalism," in G. Gorovitz, *et al.* (Eds.), *Moral Problems in Medicine*, Englewood Cliffs, N.J.: Prentice Hall, 1976, pp. 190-191.

12. G. Dworkin, "Paternalism," p. 200.

13. G. Dworkin, "Paternalism," p. 185.

14. J. Feinberg, *Social Philosophy*, p. 49. Feinberg quotes Mill here.

15. G. Dworkin, "Paternalism," p. 193.

16. Quoted by G. Dworkin in "Paternalism," p. 191.

17. D.N. MacCormick, "Rights in Legislation," in P. Hacker and J. Raz (eds.), *Law, Morality and Society: Essays in Honor of H.L.A. Hart*, Clarendon: Oxford University Press, 1977, pp. 188-209.

18. Some recent writers on these two kinds of rights include D.D. Raphael, "Human Rights, Old and New," in D.D. Raphael (ed.), *Political Theory and the Rights of Man*, Indianapolis: Indiana University Press, 1967, pp. 54-67; M. Golding, "Towards a Theory of Human Rights," *Monist*, 52, 1968, pp. 521-549; H.L.A. Hart, "Bentham on Legal Rights," in A. Simpson (ed.), *Jurisprudence*; J. Feinberg, "Voluntary Euthanasia and The Inalienable Right to Life," in *Philosophy and Public Affairs*, 7, No. 2, 1978, pp. 93-123; S. Scheffler, "Natural Rights, Equality and the Minimal State," in *The Canadian Journal of Philosophy*, 6, No. 1, 1976, pp. 64-76; F. Michelman, "Constitutional Welfare Rights and a Theory of Justice," in N. Daniels (ed.), *Reading Rawls*, New York: Basic Books, 1976, pp. 319-346. Notable is Michelman's argument that welfare rights are essential to individual self-respect. This could also apply to the patient role; R. Dworkin, *Taking Rights Seriously*, Cambridge: Harvard University Press, 1977; J. Nickel, "Are Social and Economic Rights Real Human Rights?" Paper read at Philosophy and Public Affairs Society Meeting, New York City, City University of New York Graduate Center, 1977; D.N. MacCormick, "Rights in Legislation"; F. Carney, "Is There a Moral Right to Health Care?" Paper read at Bioethics Center for Law, Washington, D.C., October 22, 1977. Carney distinguishes freedom and benefit rights. See also M.P. Golding, "Rights: A Historical Sketch," in E. and B. Bandman (eds.) *Bioethics and Human Rights*, Boston: Little, Brown, 1978, pp. 44-50. For another recent and insightful treatment of rights as rights to freedom and well being, see A. Gewirth, *Reason and Morality*, Chicago: The University of Chicago Press, 1978, pp. 63-103 and pp. 371-373.

19. E. Bandman, "Problems for Nurses in a Rights Based View of Nursing," presented at a conference on "Nursing and Humanities: A Public Dialogue," at the University of Connecticut Health Center, Farmington, Connecticut, November 11, 1977.

20. E. Bandman, "The Dilemma of Life and Death: Shall we let them die?" *Nursing Forum*, Vol. 17, No. 2, 1978, pp. 118-132.

21. M. Walzer, "Consenting to One's own death: The Case of Brutus," in M. Kohl, (ed.), *Beneficent Euthanasia*, Buffalo: N.Y.: Prometheus, 1975, pp. 100-106.

22. For an elaboration of this distinction between waiving instances of a right and relinquishing the right itself, see J. Feinberg, "Voluntary Euthanasia and 'The Inalienable Right to Life.'"

23. See J. Feinberg, "Voluntary Euthanasia and 'The Inalienable Right to Life.'"

24. R. Dworkin, *Taking Rights Seriously*, Introduction, Chapters 7, 11, 12, especially pp. xi-xii, pp. 191-193; 257-273.

25. One might compare this account, however, with S. Bok's illuminating account in *Lying: Moral Choice in Public and Private Life*, New York: Pantheon, 1978, especially pp. 238-241.

26. D.N. MacCormick, "Rights in Legislation," p. 208.

7

Moral Responsibility in Nursing*

Natalie Abrams

Ethical issues in the nursing profession have recently received increased attention.[1] One of the most important of these issues is the question of individual moral responsibility. The importance of this issue is emphasized by the following written statements on nursing practice: "The attending physician, and, to a more limited degree, the medical resident and intern function as individuals and are individually responsible for their actions. The employees of the hospital, even professional nurses, are agents of the institution and in that capacity are obligated to report and to record their activities. Therein lies one of the dilemmas of nursing."[2] "To be a nurse requires the willing assumption of ethical responsibility in every dimension of practice."[3] This latter quote is the opening statement of a special feature on ethics in the May, 1977 issue of the *American Journal of Nursing*.

The present trend to encourage the professionalization of nursing and the assumption of more individual responsibility can be interpreted in a number of different ways in accordance with the different meanings of the word "responsible."[4] For example, someone can be said to be a responsible person, the kind of person one could trust. Respon-

*I would like to thank Joseph M. Healey, Jr., J.D., and John Troyer, Ph.D., for very helpful comments on a first draft of this chapter.

sibility in this sense is a character trait and certainly urging nurses, or anyone, to be responsible in this sense is nothing new. One could also be responsible for performing certain kinds of tasks. For example, one could be responsible for "people," as exemplified in the statement "she is my responsibility now." One could be responsible for events, as in the statement "arranging for discharge is my responsibility." One could be responsible for certain behavior, as in "my responsibility is to put in that IV." One might even be said to be responsible for "objects," as in the statement "the ward is my responsibility." Frequently, nursing responsibility is conceptualized in terms of time and space, i.e., in terms of a particular unit for a certain period of time. Although defining the limits of nursing practice is certainly an important and pressing issue, I do not believe that this interpretation of responsibility in terms of duties captures what is meant by urging nurses to exercise more autonomy and to assume more responsibility. The assumption of moral responsibility usually refers to a willingness to act on one's moral beliefs and to accept accountability for one's actions. It is this latter notion of responsibility that I believe is being recommended by the nursing profession and it is this notion of responsibility which is called into question in certain situations in hospital nursing practice.

The following chapter is an attempt to analyze specific situations in hospital nursing practice which pose "moral dilemmas," and therefore highlight the issue of individual responsibility. I suggest that there are similarities between assuming moral responsibility in those situations in which there is a moral dilemma, what I call "professional non-compliance," and civil disobedience.

A presupposition of the chapter is that the situations of hospital nursing practice which best pose the issue of individual moral responsibility, in the sense of a willingness to act on one's beliefs and to accept accountability for one's actions, are those situations which include reference to the nurse's place in the social structure of the hospital and to the nurse's role in decision making. Furthermore, such situations involve basic disagreements between the nurse and some other primary decision maker, whether it be a physician or any rank, a nursing superior, an administrator, or even the patient. This presupposition is not meant to imply, however, that such disagreements are the sole source of ethical issues confronting the nurse. The traditional ethical questions in health care are certainly as significant for the nurse as for the physician (here I am referring to such issues as euthanasia, abortion, experimentation, distribution of health care, truth-telling, and so on). However, the arguments per se about these issues appear to be the same, regardless of to whom they are directed. More importantly, in terms of the focus of this chapter on individual responsibility, the interesting and unique issues facing nurses include reference to the nurse's particular position in regard to decision making within the social and hierarchical structure of the hospital. [5]

It is for this reason that I am focusing on these situations and ethical issues in nursing practice, rather than the traditional questions as seen from the point of view of the nurse. I assume, in fact, that there is no such thing as "the nurse" or "the nurse's point of view." There is, rather, a group of individual people with different moral points of view who happen to occupy the same position in a social and professional setting. The only acceptable approach, therefore, to understanding ethical issues as they confront the nurse is to focus on the common factors which warrant that title. Obviously, this requires that one focus on the nurse as an occupant of a particular role in a social setting.

AREAS OF DISAGREEMENT BETWEEN THE NURSE AND OTHER HEALTH PROFESSIONALS

There appear to be three basic areas of potential disagreement between a nurse and other health professionals, although, undoubtedly, many other areas of possible disagreement could be found. One possible area of disagreement concerns the so-called health "facts" or "judgments" about a case, i.e., the nurse may agree or disagree with other decision makers concerning the patient's health status. For example, there might be either agreement or disagreement concerning the diagnosis or evaluation of the patient's physical condition, the optimum treatment, the expected reaction from a particular procedure, the risk to a patient from a certain procedure, the prognosis for the patient's illness, or even the physical or psychological effect on the patient of telling him about his illness. I am presupposing here that fully trained and experienced nurses do have professional judgments about such issues and that, given their expertise and growing knowledge, it is not acceptable to discount their judgments in these matters. Whether their judgments in any given case ultimately turn out to be right or wrong is not the point. As opposed to the layman who may have opinions with little or no knowledge base, the nurse's background compels consideration, at the least, of his or her professional judgment.

A second area of possible disagreement concerns the basic moral issues presented by a case. For example, a nurse may agree or disagree with other decision makers over such issues as whether or not a patient has a right to certain information, whether family members have rights, whether confidentiality can ever be broken, and, if so, when, and whether a certain risk/benefit ratio is acceptable.

A third area of possible disagreement concerns the relative importance of moral versus health concerns. In other words, even though there may be agreement concerning the health-related issues involved in a case, as well as the basic moral issues involved, there may not be agreement over whether health or moral concerns should receive priority. This, in turn, can lead to disagreement over the actual decision to be made in a given case. It might be successfully argued that a belief that either moral or health concerns are of more importance is itself a moral claim, such that if there is disagreement over this issue, there can be said to be disagreement over a basic moral issue. Although this appears to me to be a forceful argument, for the present purposes of identifying basic areas of possible disagreement, I believe it is best to keep this distinction separate.

Underlying all of these areas of possible disagreement is whether or not the nurse places any value on functioning within the existing system. In other words, does the nurse accept or reject the system's underlying principles and objectives. For the purposes of this chapter, a "moral dilemma" is being defined as a situation in which a nurse has to make an actual decision in the face of a disagreement with a health professional of higher rank *and* in which the nurse does in fact place some value on functioning within the existing system and would therefore find it morally troublesome to disobey. The moral dilemma results from the existence of two factors: first, a disagreement between the nurse and another health professional about the correct moral position and/or about the correct approach to the patient's health; and, secondly, the nurse's desire to function within the existing health-care structure. On the other hand, if the nurse does not accept the general principles of the existing health-care establishment and therefore does not place any value on working within its structure, the nurse is not confronted with a moral dilemma in the sense of an inner conflict about what course of action should or should not be followed, although such a situation does undoubtedly pose many practical problems.

The existence of a moral dilemma can be perhaps best understood by examining a sample situation. For example, if a nurse and physician are in agreement about the health status of a patient but the physician believes patients do not have the right to information about their illnesses, whereas the nurse believes they do, the nurse is confronted with the decision as to whether to go along with the physician and withhold information or to follow his or her own beliefs. On the one hand, if the nurse basically disapproves of the existing health-care system and sees no value in supporting it, the nurse would not be faced with a moral dilemma, i.e., it would be clear to the nurse that the correct course of action would be to inform the patient about his or her condition. It should not be *morally* problematic for the nurse to go against the physician's position by telling the patient. Here, there might seem to be a conflict between a moral value and a desire or personal interest, perhaps in not losing one's job. However, there would not seem to be a moral dilemma in terms of a difficulty for the nurse to decide what he or she *should* do. On the other hand, if the nurse basically approves of the existing hierarchical structure and its underlying principles, the nurse is confronted with a moral dilemma in the sense of not knowing which course of action should actually be followed. There is a moral dilemma between two conflicting beliefs both of which the nurse holds to be of prima facie value, telling the patient and acting within the system. It is the existence of these two opposing factors which makes the situation morally problematic for the nurse and which defines at least one type of moral dilemma.

MORAL RESPONSIBILITY
AND CIVIL DISOBEDIENCE

I would like to suggest some similarities between assuming moral responsibility in those situations in which there is a moral dilemma as
defined, what I shall call professional non-compliance, and civil disobedience. Again, situations posing moral dilemmas are those in
which the course of action approved by the nurse differs from that
approved by a health professional of higher rank and yet the nurse
places some value on acting within the existing system because he or
she accepts its underlying principles.

Of central importance is the fact that in cases of both civil disobedience and professional non-compliance, there is an existing authoritarian structure which is thought to be legitimate, yet a disagreement over
a particular issue or decision. (Here I am basically following Rawls'
definition of civil disobedience.)[6] Although some value is seen in
obeying the system, a particular decision of the system is considered,
by an individual, to be sufficiently against the underlying principles to
warrant disobedience. A second point of similarity is the following.
The individual who performs an act of civil disobedience "invokes the
commonly shared conception of justice"[7] of the community; similarly,
a nurse in a situation of moral dilemma who refuses to obey a superior's orders may be able to appeal to commonly shared principles
that underlie the hospital structure and the professional roles of both
nurse and physician. In neither case does the individual appeal solely
to his or her own set of moral or religious precepts, although these
may coincide with and support one's claims. Rather, the appeal is
being made to the set of principles that everyone involved purportedly
accepts. Essentially, then, the charge is being made that the law or
order which is being rejected violates the underlying principles on
which the law or order itself is based. This points out a distinction
between what Rawls calls an act of civil disobedience and one of "conscientious refusal."[8] In the latter case, an individual appeals to his or
her own moral principles or individual conscience. There is no commonly shared ground or set of principles to which the individual
appeals. In cases of conscientious refusal, therefore, the problem exists

of justifying individual conscience as a guide to action, an especially difficult problem when there is a clash between two individual consciences or between that of an individual and a collective, as expressed in law. However, it should be noted that justifying conscience as a guide to action is also necessary even in those situations in which there is no clash between two individual consciences or between that of an individual and a collective. Justifying conscience as a guide to action is necessary even in those situations in which one obeys. Otherwise, one is committed to the position that when people obey laws or authority they are acting against their consciences. Surely, conscientious action does not occur only when one goes against a law. One can also act in good conscience when one obeys.

Although this distinction between civil disobedience or professional non-compliance and conscientious refusal may be difficult to make in practice, it is a very important distinction, for if disagreement between nurse and physician or other decision maker is seen as similar to conscientious refusal rather than to civil disobedience, the disagreement can be reduced simply to concerns over individual moral judgments, with no possible hope for a solution except in terms of a power struggle. If, on the other hand, the nurse's disagreement can be interpreted as a claim, e.g., that the physician has not respected and acted upon one of the principles which the physician has implicitly or explicitly accepted, there can be some attempt at a mutually agreeable solution.

The underlying principles or commonly shared beliefs in cases of civil disobedience would be those expressed in the Constitution, such as equal protection and due process. The underlying principles or shared set of values in the hospital context would be those general beliefs shared by the nursing and medical professions, as well as the hospital administration. Principles such as always acting in the best interest of the patient, protecting confidentiality, obtaining informed consent for experimental procedures, obtaining consultations when believed necessary, and even respecting the scientific method are just a few examples of the kinds of principles which nurses, physicians, hospital administrators, and most patients would accept. These principles can be seen as serving a function somewhat similar to that of the Constitution. Although there can be considerable disagreement concerning their implementation, there is often agreement about the basic principles against which individual actions can be judged. In theory at least, if such underlying beliefs are agreed to by all, conflict resolution should not be a power struggle but rather an appeal to and an interpretation of these basic ideas.

It might be argued that agreement in principle without agreement in practice is of no value, and also that the principles underlying the health-care professions and the rules governing their implementation are not as explicit or formal as those of the Constitution.[9] While disputes over the implementation of particular principles do pose serious problems, the situation with the Constitution, however, is quite similar. Despite agreement over the principles of equality, justice, due process, and liberty, there is enormous disagreement over which policies do in fact respect or violate these principles. The battles over affirmative action as exemplified by the Bakke suit, and over the practical implications of the equal rights amendment are cases in point. Underlying principles, however, provide at least the basis for equitable and consistent decision making. Without such principles, there is no hope for decision making to be anything other than a series of arbitrary ad hoc rules and regulations. Furthermore, many conflicts in the hospital context do not involve disagreement over the principles themselves or even their implementation, but rather involve a decision maker's conscious refusal or unconscious failure to act on principle. In such situations, the goal would be to convince the individual in question that acting on principles is required by the standards of his or her profession.

Another similarity between civil disobedience and professional non-compliance is that just as acts of civil disobedience are always done in public and not covertly, the same should be true of acts of professional non-compliance. There should be no attempt to disobey and hope that no one will discover what has been done. Obviously, what is missing in the hospital context is the equivalent to a judicial system which can review the particular legislation in terms of constitutional principles. Such a review body within the hospital, however, would not seem to be an unrealistic proposal in light of pressure for the health-care professions, especially the medical profession, to institute measures for peer review.

Four additional constraints might also be placed on acts of what is being called professional non-compliance in accord with Rawls' constraints on civil disobedience. First, if such non-compliance is based on an appeal to a widely accepted set of professional standards, it should be limited to instances of significant violation. Second, normal appeals to those in authority should already have been made. Before refusing to comply with a directive, it is incumbent upon the nurse to discuss the issue with the appropriate person. Professional non-compliance should be used only as a last resort and only in ways so that it is not misunderstood. Third, certain instances of civil disobedience or professional non-compliance are clearly not justified. They constitute those instances in which disobedience itself violates an important underlying principle. In the hospital context, non-compliance in an emergency or surgical setting could lead to placing a patient at greater risk. Under those circumstances disobedience would not be permissible. Fourth, if an individual does perform an act of professional non-compliance, he or she must receive the appropriate sanctions. Arguments to the contrary would essentially be claiming either that the individual did not disobey existing law or orders or that the individual could privately decide to disobey because one's conscience directed him to do so. However, "no law could be written which would simultaneously grant any citizen the right to exempt himself from its jurisdiction...clearly such laws would be self-nullifying."[10] Similarly, with regard to nursing, those who choose to disobey orders cannot refuse sanctions, for in acts of civil disobedience, "the law is broken, but fidelity to law is expressed...by the willingness to accept the legal consequences of one's conduct."[11]

Claiming that professional non-compliance is justifiable or permissible is quite different from claiming that it is required or obligatory. To claim that it is obligatory would be to claim that the nurse must refuse compliance with a directive which he or she believes is not in accordance with the basic principles of the health-care professions. If it were obligatory, however, it would have to be a duty of the nurse —as a nurse per se, as an employee of the institution, or as an individual person. Since refusing compliance brings with it a great risk of personal sacrifice, possibly in terms of losing one's job, I would like to suggest that such an action should be seen as supererogatory, loosely defined as beyond the call of duty. Such an action could not be part of one's duty as a professional nurse or as an employee of an institution and also possibly result in loss of one's job. In principle at least, one cannot risk losing his job in the course of performing his duty. At best, an act of non-compliance could be seen as one's duty as an individual person.

The above discussion is most applicable to those situations of moral dilemma in which the disagreement arises over a moral issue itself or over the ranking of moral versus health criteria, which, as noted before, can also be viewed as a moral conflict. However, I believe it can also be applied to those situations in which the moral dilemma arises over a conflict concerning the health-related judgments involved in a case, although clearly this is a harder claim to support. The basic underlying principles to which an individual can appeal in situations of civil disobedience or professional non-compliance can be of four different types. First, there are legal principles. Any appeal to these principles could be seen as a case of civil disobedience in the ordinary sense. Second, there are professional standards of conduct. These are the ones, e.g., of confidentiality, informed consent, which constitute the basic principles to which I have already referred and to which appeal would be made in the case of a moral disagreement. Third, there are moral standards which are not included within a professional code. It might be possible to argue that a physician and nurse are members of a moral community, as well as a profession, and therefore one might appeal to the community's moral standards in evaluating a particular decision. This is a much more difficult approach and would have to be carefully conceptualized. Fourth, there are the standards of the health sciences. It is these standards which can be appealed to in a dispute over the health-related judgments of a case. Two different claims can operate in such a disagreement. The nurse, e.g., can believe that the physician is incorrectly judging the situation because of a disregard for evidence, which would clearly constitute a violation of a professional principle. Alternatively, the nurse can simply interpret the evidence differently. This would not constitute violation of a standard, but it is exactly this issue which would have to be decided by a review body. Essentially, then, disagreement in a moral dilemma over the health-related issues of the case might also be viewed as the basis for professional non-compliance, in the sense that the individual is appealing to accepted principles.

Similarities between civil disobedience and professional non-compliance are thus applicable to cases of moral dilemma in which the underlying principles of the system are respected. Situations in which the underlying principles are not respected, however, are entirely different. In such situations, the nurse rejects the system itself. These cases are somewhat similar to what Rawls calls those of "militancy." Here "the basic structure is thought to be so unjust or else to depart so widely from its own professional ideals that one must try to prepare the way for radical or even revolutionary change."[12] Acts of civil disobedience or professional non-compliance are not appropriate in such situations, since the underlying principles themselves or the process itself is rejected. A much more radical type of non-compliance might be justified or even seen as necessary in such a situation. It is essential, therefore, for the individual nurse, as well as the nursing profession, to evaluate cases of disagreement in order to determine exactly what is at issue or what is under dispute. It is only following such an evaluation that it would be possible to determine the appropriate response. It is impossible for a nurse to assume "individual moral responsibility" and determine the appropriate conduct without an adequate understanding of the source of the moral dilemma.

NOTES

1. For the purposes of this chapter, the terms "ethical" and "moral" are assumed to be equivalent in meaning and are used interchangeably.

2. Mauksch, Hans O., "The Organizational Context of Nursing Practice," in *The Nursing Profession: Five Sociological Essays*, Fred Dairs (ed.), Wiley and Sons, Inc.: New York, 1966, p. 113.

3. Levine, Myra E., "Nursing Ethics and the Ethical Nurse," *American Journal of Nursing*, May, 1977, p. 845.

4. For a fuller discussion of these meanings of responsibility, see Becker, Lawrence C., *On Justifying Moral Judgments*, Humanities Press: New York, 1973, especially chapter XIII, pp. 128-140.

5. Restricting my consideration to hospital-based situations should not be taken to imply the primacy of the hospital context over other very interesting and difficult settings in which nurses function. Time and space simply demand some restrictions.

6. Rawls, John, *A Theory of Justice*, Harvard University Press; Massachusetts, 1971, especially pp. 363-395. I thank John Troyer for pointing out that Rawls' theory of civil disobedience is considerably different from Thoreau's view in his *Civil Disobedience* and from Gandhi's "passive resistance" movement. The similarities which are noted between civil disobedience and professional non-compliance therefore do not necessarily follow from these other theories of civil disobedience.

7. *Ibid.*, p. 365.

8. *Ibid.*, p. 368.

9. I thank Joseph M. Healey for pointing out this argument.

10. Earle, William, "Private Conscience or Myself as Hero," in *Conscientious Actions, the Revelation of the Pentagon Papers*, Peter A. French (ed.), Schenkman Pub. Co.: Massachusetts, 1974, p. 17.

11. Rawls, *op. cit.*, p. 366.

12. *Ibid.*, pp. 367-368.

Some Reflections on Authority and the Nurse

John Ladd

As is evident from the chapters in this volume, there are a number of different problems confronting nurses collectively and individually. In this chapter, I want to focus on some of the moral quandaries faced by nurses that originate in what Touster calls the "complex and compelling system of authority which inhibits independence and transforms that moral character of her work largely into questions of obedience, disobedience, or evasion of authority."[1] I use the term "quandary" advisedly, because I want to stress the connotation of a "subjective perception" of the dilemma.[2] For, although many of the problems connected with authority appear to be moral dilemmas, strictly speaking, they are not really dilemmas at all and should therefore, for logical and ethical reasons, be handled quite differently from dilemmas.[3] If we try to clarify some logical and ethical aspects of the concept of authority, especially as it relates to nursing, we may make some headway in determining where the real issues lie and how to approach them.

First, a few comments are in order concerning what I shall call the *social issues* relating to nursing, namely, all those problems connected with the generally inferior social and economic status assigned to nurses in the medical hierarchy. As Touster and others have pointed out, present-day oppression and exploitation of nurses can, in large measure, be explained historically, for, in the past, nurses generally belonged to the lower social and economic classes and have almost always been women. When viewed sociologically, these facts may explain why in nursing circles today there is so much emphasis on the conception of nursing as a profession; by becoming professionals, nurses will be able to enter the middle class and so achieve social parity with other middle-class professionals, including doctors.[4]

For obvious reasons, these social problems loom large in the consciousness of nurses and of women in general. But there is not much that a philosopher can do about oppression and exploitation, whether it be economic or sexist, except to deplore it. We should not forget, however, that things are changing. Our age is an age of revolutions, not merely political revolutions, but biological, technological, social, and sexual revolutions. The winds of change are upon us and there is no reason to believe that the social, economic, and sexist status of nurses will remain the same as it has been in the past.

These revolutions, like all revolutions, also create many ethical problems that are interesting and that are enormously complex and troublesome: e.g., questions like how much of the old to cast away and how much to retain? What methods can and should be used to secure the necessary changes? What should be the long-range goals as contrasted with the short-range goals? These questions are already incorporated into public debates over such things as reverse-discrimination, fair employment practices, and unionization.

Let us suppose, however, that as a result of revolutions of this type the social issues connected with nursing are resolved, or at least transformed so radically that it will no longer be true that being a nurse means being female, uneducated, and lower class, or that being a doctor means being male, educated, and upper class. Other important ethical problems encountered by nurses would still remain to be resolved, in particular, ethical problems relating to authority and role differentiation. These problems were aired by Plato a long time ago, quite independently of the particular social issues that nurses are concerned with today. We should not forget that Plato was one of the first philosophers to advocate the equality of the sexes and that although he firmly believed in authority and role differentiation, he certainly did not believe in male domination. Authoritarianism is not necessarily sexist or economically exploitative.

AUTHORITY AND POWER

Any discussion of authority—including the authority of doctors, hospital administrators, head nurses, deans, judges, and generals—must begin by distinguishing between power and authority. Authority always carries the connotation of legitimacy, which power does not. Following de Jouvenal, I shall define "power" as the "capacity to make oneself obeyed," that is, the capacity to make others do what one wants them to do against their own desires and preferences and against their will.[5] There is no question that individual physicians and organizations, such as hospitals, wield a great deal of power, or "clout," and that nurses, as well as patients, are often "forced" to do things or to suffer things that they would prefer, often with good reason, not to do or not to suffer. How to respond to power when it is illegitimate, illegal, or immoral raises many interesting ethical questions, but they are of a different sort from questions about how to respond to authority. Here Touster's term "evasion" seems entirely appropriate: if someone sticks a gun in your ribs, either literally or figuratively, evasion is an entirely appropriate response. If, therefore, the alleged authority of physicians and hospital managers is simply a matter of power, then the moral principles governing a nurse's or a patient's proper responses to their orders would not differ essentially from the principles that mandate a person's responses to the orders of one of his captors in, say, a concentration camp: that is, subterfuge, escape, resistance, and sabotage.

But we are not concerned here with power as such—which need not be, and often is not, legitimate—but with authority in the sense that it connotes legitimacy. Although "authority" is sometimes defined as "legitimate power," or, if you wish, as "legal power" or "morally justified power," in order to avoid confusion, it is better to regard power as an adjunct of authority or a consequence of authority rather than as definitive of it. After all, Plato found no need for power in his republic; the authority of the philosopher-king was founded on reason, not on power. Let us therefore try to analyze the concept of authority without reference to the concept of power.

The best way to understand the concept of authority is to approach it from the point of view of the individual who is subject to it. Authority calls for respect rather than fear. Respect for authority, in turn, implies the right to command rather than the power to coerce. For, in Hart's words, "to command is characteristically to exercise authority over men, not power to inflict harm, and though it may be combined with threats of harm a command is primarily an appeal not to fear but to respect for authority."[6]

Insofar as authority is based on respect rather than on fear, it is something that is accepted voluntarily; the acceptance of authority implies a willingness to comply with the commands of authority on the part of the subject. The authority commands, and the subject obeys, because, for one reason or another, he acknowledges that the authority has the right to command and that he or she, on that account, has the duty to obey. Thus, de Jouvenal says: "To follow authority is a voluntary act. Authority ends where voluntary assent ends."[7]

It is assumed that the subject is willing to comply with the commands of an authority even when the particular acts demanded are contrary to his or her own personal wishes, desires, or interests. In addition, the subject obeys the command not because of its content or because it is rational, but simply because it is commanded by an authority that he or she has accepted.[8] In other words, authority is to be obeyed not because what it commands is reasonable, but because it is reasonable to obey its commands. In this sense, the *ipse dixits* of an authority serve *eo ipso* as binding reasons for a person to do or to refrain from doing something. For this reason, authority is often said to imply the "voluntary surrender of judgment" or the "voluntary abdication of choice" on the part of the subject in the area over which the authority rules.[9]

However, it should be observed that, strictly speaking, assent, i.e. acceptance, is by itself neither sufficient nor necessary to make a person an authority over others; it is possible for people to *think* that they ought to obey a person who actually has no right to command them, just as it is also possible for people to *think* that they need not obey a person who actually does have such a right. If the authority is legitimate, then it is more nearly accurate to say that people subject to it *ought* to accept the authority, that is, ought to assent to its right to command, and so *ought* to obey its commands.

To say that people ought to accept an authority and to obey its commands means that there is a good reason for them to do so. But there is no good reason for people to accept and obey an authority if the authority claimed has no basis; the claim that a person has the right to command others must have a basis or ground. As with rights in general, if the right to command has no basis, then there is no reason for accepting and obeying what is claimed to be an authority. Hence, if the claimant is unable to provide the kind of validation or justification required of authority, the claim to authority falls to the ground; it has no logical or moral force.[10] It follows that the *burden of proof* lies on the claimant to show that the authority claimed is legitimate, rather than on those over whom the authority is claimed; the latter are not obliged to provide their own counterarguments against the claim of authority.[11]

SPURIOUS AUTHORITIES AND THE LIMITS TO AUTHORITY

It is impossible to understand what is at issue in many of the ethical problems relating to authority and nursing, unless we take into consideration that, in many cases, people do not really have the authority that they claim to have. Let us call such persons *spurious authorities* (or "false authorities"). As I have already pointed out, there is no valid reason, much less a moral reason, for accepting a spurious authority; if the authority is spurious, one has no moral obligation to comply with his commands and one should not feel "guilty" about not doing so. Therefore, whether or not to comply with the demands of a spurious authority does not, strictly speaking, present a moral dilemma, that is, a situation in which one is forced to choose between conflicting duties.[12]

It should also be pointed out that there are always limits to the scope of an authority, not only limits as regards those over whom it has jurisdiction, but also as regards the kind of conduct that it may command. With the possible exception of the Almighty, there is no such thing as an unlimited authority; that is, the right of one person to command is always restricted to one group of people, one sphere of action, in short, to one specific context.[13] Thus, granting that a physician has a certain kind of authority over, say, a nurse or a patient, that authority does not extend over everything conceivable that the nurse or the patient might do or wish to do.[14] If a person tries to command others who do not come under his or her authority, or tries to command them in matters that do not come under that authority, that person is said to "exceed his or her authority." Based on what I have already said, it thus follows that no one has the duty to obey the commands of a person when that person exceeds his or her authority. The limits of an authority are part and parcel of the validation (or justification) of authority, since the limits of one's obligation to obey have the same basis as the obligation to accept and obey.[15]

By now, the intent of my argument should be clear. The duty of a nurse to comply with the orders of a doctor or administrator depends on the nature, source, and limits of that person's authority. If that authority is spurious, or the orders exceed the person's authority, the nurse may be in a quandary. However, there is no moral dilemma. Although it may be prudent to comply with a doctor's or administrator's order because he has power, it is not ethically necessary to justify noncompliance as such. In other words, it is not necessary for a nurse to "think up" a special reason for not complying with an order such as that it is morally wrong: for example, to lie to a patient. Ethically, the correct response to the order to lie to a patient is either that the doctor has no right to tell the nurse what to do—i.e., the doctor has no authority—or that the doctor has no right to tell the nurse to do that particular thing—i.e., he has exceeded his authority. In other words, the nurse is not required to defend her refusal with a counterargument, for example, to the effect that she has a duty to the patient that conflicts with her duty to the doctor. For, in such cases, she has no duty to the doctor at all.[16]

BASES OF AUTHORITY

In investigating the basis of authority in medicine—whether it be the authority of the physician, of the hospital administrator, or of whomever else—over other persons, say, nurses or patients, we must recognize at the very outset that the issues are complicated and that the relationships in question may involve many different kinds of authority. But we should be careful not to allow the complexity of the relationships to conceal the spuriousness of some claims to authority on the part of doctors or other professionals in the health-care system. Once again, it should not be forgotten that the burden of proof always falls on the doctor, hospital administrator, or whoever else makes the authority claim. Ethically, then, it is always proper to respond to an order by asking: Why should I obey you? What is the basis of your authority?[17]

There are, of course, many different bases of authority and, accordingly, many different kinds of authority. In order to determine what grounds there might be for authority in medicine, say, the authority of the doctor over a nurse or over a patient, let us examine some possible answers to the question: Why should we obey A., an authority?

Let us start with the distinction between authorities for *beliefs* and authorities over *conduct*. By the former, which might be called "intellectual" or "cognitive" authority, I mean the kind of authority that is used to establish the truth of some proposition or other. Technically, an argument that uses authority in this way is called "an argument from authority." An argument from authority is based on the general principle that if one has good reason to believe that A. knows *p* and asserts *p*, then one has a sufficiently good reason to believe *p* oneself—on A.'s word, so to speak. It is often highly reasonable to "take the word" of someone who knows something better than we do, e.g., the word of an expert who has specialized technical knowledge that we do not possess. The authority of the doctor is often this type of intellectual authority, the authority of an expert, whose word we readily take, as to what is ailing us, because it is in our own interest to do so. But it is not self-evident that this kind of authority makes the physician an authority over conduct.

It has often been maintained that a person who has specialized knowledge—i.e., who is an authority in the intellectual sense—automatically has authority over conduct or practical authority—e.g., the right to command. This is the position taken in Plato's *Republic*. The rulers in the Republic have special knowledge on how to rule; therefore, they have the right to rule and others have the duty to obey. Their intellectual qualifications, as experts in ruling, *eo ipso* make them into authorities over conduct, or practical authorities. Doctors are sometimes thought to have authority over conduct for the same sort of reason. However, before the transition from authority in the intellectual sense to authority in the practical sense—i.e., over conduct—can be considered valid, some additional theoretical underpinning is needed. In Plato's case, the transition is justified by reference to his twofold doctrine that knowledge is virtue and that ethical knowledge is a *techne*—i.e., the kind of knowledge possessed by experts. There are, of course, serious philosophical objections to both doctrines.[18] But in any case, it is far from obvious that doctors possess the kind of knowledge and virtue required of rulers in Plato's Republic.

It hardly seems necessary to dwell on the absurdity of the idea that intellectual authority automatically gives a person the right to order people around. There is nothing extraordinary about the fact that we have to rely on others for specialized information of various sorts, and that we have to accept what they say on authority. But, at that, it still is possible for an individual to decide what to do and what not to do, based on the authoritative information that he or she has received from others. It is obvious that in dealing with scientific matters, it is almost always necessary to take the word of expert authorities. But in this regard, medical science is ostensibly no different from, say, physics and engineering. No one who is an authority in one of these fields thereby acquires the authority to make decisions for other people. As I have already suggested, anyone who wishes to base a doctor's right to command on his superior knowledge must be prepared to *show* that doctors know more about (medical?) ethics than others and are more virtuous than their nurses or their patients.[19]

BASES OF AUTHORITY:
LEGITIMATION AND VALIDATION

Let us now turn to authority over conduct, i.e., the kind of practical authority that generates the obligation to accept and obey orders on the part of persons subject to it. As I have already remarked, authority in this sense requires the abdication of choice with regard to what a subject does or does not do. The question before us is: by what right does one person require someone else's abdication of choice?

Before trying to answer this question we should note that not all authority has or needs a moral basis. There are many kinds of activities that require authority but that are not moral activities per se. Consequently, we must allow for other types of legitimation and validation besides moral justification.

If we take a broad look at authority, we see a great variety of activities that require authorities of one sort or another: for example, authorities are needed in playing games, e.g., captains of teams and umpires; for running orderly meetings, e.g., chairpersons; for operating businesses, e.g., managers; and so on. Employer-employee relations almost always involve some kind of authority of the employer over the employee.

From these considerations, it follows that some legitimate authorities do not need a moral basis and that consequently not all obligations to accept and obey an authority are moral obligations. For it should be obvious that different bases generate different kinds of obligations on the part of those affected. For example, if the authority has only a legal basis, then it will generate only a legal obligation, unless we assume that every legal obligation is also a moral obligation.[20]

The issues involved here will be easier to discuss if we break down the question about the basis of authority into two separate questions: Why is authority needed, i.e., what makes it legitimate? And, why should an individual accept and comply with a particular authority? Although for the purpose of this chapter we need to keep these questions separate, it will become clear that when we take up the ethical issues relating to authority they tend to become indistinguishable. It will be convenient to refer to the process of establishing the legitimacy of an authority as *legitimation* and the process of establishing the obligation to accept and obey an authority as *validation*.[21] Let us begin with legitimation.

Turning to modes of legitimation, we should note that many authorities acquire their legitimacy on the ground that they fill an essential need. Thus, organizations generally need authorities in order to operate efficiently: the authority coordinates, organizes, and plans, while others are expected to acknowledge this authority and to comply with the orders. Let us call the kind of authority that is adopted for the sake of efficiency *organizational authority*. Formal organizations of all kinds, including health-care bureaucracies and hospitals, involve organizational authority of a special sort, namely, a hierarchy of authorities.

Questions about the legitimacy of particular organizational authorities generally revolve around their so-called rationality, that is, their efficiency and effectiveness in promoting a goal and the worthiness of the goal itself. Assuming that one of the goals of a hospital is to provide treatment facilities, then its managerial structure, i.e., the structure of authority, might be legitimized in terms of its ability to facilitate this goal.

Among goals that may be used to legitimize organizational authority, some may be moral, some may be nonmoral, and some may be downright immoral. Activities such as games may be subsumed under nonmoral types. Organized crime and totalitarian organizations exemplify the immoral type.

For our purposes, only the first two kinds of organized activities are of interest. Let us assume that the health-care authorities we are concerned with do not fall under the category of organized crime.

Let us now turn to the second question: why should a person accept and comply with the orders of an authority? In particular, why obey the captain, the chairperson, or the boss? Disregarding questions of incentives and disincentives, i.e., rewards and sanctions that proceed from power rather than from authority, we are really concerned here with finding good reasons for accepting and complying with the commands of an authority as such.

In the case of organizational authority, which is our concern here, it is often easy to answer these questions. For example, in games and in meetings, it is reasonable to comply with the commands of the authority because doing so makes the activity in which one is participating more efficient and effective. Here, the motive or ground for accepting the authority in question is the acceptance of the goal, and the recognition that a particular authority structure is a means to that goal. In Kant's words, to will the end is to will the means.

Sometimes, one shares the goal with others, in particular, with the person who is the authority. In that case, we have validation based on participation: sharing the goal. On the other hand, there are cases in which the person subject to an authority does not share the goals that legitimize that authority. When goals diverge, compliance seems to be less voluntary than when they converge. Therefore, divergence requires some kind of extraneous validation. Much of the logic of authority, that is, of validation, hinges on whether there is a convergence or a divergence of goals.

CAN AUTHORITY HAVE A MORAL BASE?

Up to this point we have examined the bases of authority independently of their moral implications. It is obvious that many kinds of activities require the acceptance of an authority where moral considerations are irrelevant, peripheral, or adventitious. But, it is time to turn to a more direct consideration of the ethical aspects of legitimation and validation, which might be called the moral justification of an authority and of compliance with that authority. So far, the analysis has been in terms of what Kant called a "hypothetical imperative." We must now examine these questions from the point of view of ethics, that is, in terms of the categorical imperative.

Moral justification is distinguished from nonmoral legitimation and validation in that moral requirements take precedence over other sorts of requirements. Morality in general consists of a set of standards and principles that take precedence over other systems of rules and other enterprises, and that can be used to criticize, judge, and evaluate these other systems of rules and enterprises.[23]

We may begin with two simple and obvious kinds of justification that fit a large number of cases in which the acceptance of authority and obedience are morally required—namely, those based on contract, e.g., a contract of employment, and those established by law, e.g., the authority of a police officer, judge, or tax collector.[24]

I shall call the moral justification involved here *extrinsic justification*, because it depends on extrinsic factors, e.g., the making of a contract or a law. Without the contractual or the legislative act that creates the obligation, there would be no obligation and obedience would not be morally binding.

It should be noted that these two types of extrinsic justifications generally presuppose that the individual bound thereby does not share the goals of the authority structure. That is, they involve cases in which goals diverge. Industrial organizations provide good examples, for those subject to the authority of management and the foreman are bound to obey them by virtue of a contract of employment and not because they expect to share in the profits of the organization.

Without wishing to prejudge the issue, we might ask at this point whether the authority of a doctor over a nurse is just one of these two kinds. Is the obligation to obey simply based on contract or on law? Obviously the answer is: sometimes, but not always. A nurse, like any employee, is bound by the terms of a contract and, like other citizens, is bound to observe the law. But there may be other reasons for accepting medical authority. Let us consider what they might be.

Before proceeding, it should be observed that neither contracts nor law can require persons to do anything immoral. There are limits to contracts and limits to law, in theory at least. The nurse's moral integrity and her moral responsibilities to the patient as a person set limits to what may be required by contracts or law. An implied condition, e.g., of a contract, from a moral point of view, is that one not be required to deceive or abandon the helpless.

Apart from legitimation and validation, on the one hand, and extrinsic moral justification on the other hand, can the authority structure in medicine and nursing be morally justified? One answer might be that authority is morally justifiable if it serves a moral purpose, a morally worthy goal. Such might be the utilitarian answer.

The complexities are immediately apparent. What is the goal of medicine or of the health-care system? Is there a single, comprehensive goal of such determinateness that it could be used to justify the right of certain persons, e.g., doctors, to exercise authority over others?

Let us grant that in certain contexts authority is needed and is morally desirable—for example, in the operating room. In an operating room, the authority of the surgeon might be likened to the authority of the conductor of an orchestra: the surgeon is the chief performer and the one who "orchestrates" the proceeding. Let us grant that the aim of the procedure is to save the patient's life, i.e., a morally worthy goal. But here, as with the orchestra, we are dealing with a precisely defined, limited enterprise involving goals that we may assume are shared by all the parties involved, or, perhaps, to be more nearly accurate, we should say that they ought to be shared by all of them.

The fact is, however, that when we examine other contexts and other health-care activities, the goals are not that simply defined. In fact, there is a multiplicity of divergent goals: the doctor may be concerned to cure, the nurse may want to help the patient to adjust, and the patient may be principally worried about how to pay for everything. The divergence of goals among parties in the health-care setting accounts for the fact that there is a great deal of noncompliance and evasion, e.g., in hospitals, since it undermines the rational underpinning of the authority structure insofar as it is founded on voluntary participation.

In closing, I would like to suggest that our society relies too much on authoritarian structures to organize cooperative activities. Authoritarian structures depend for their legitimacy and effectiveness on common agreement about goals and methods. This kind of agreement is not universally found in the present-day health-care situation. It is not found in many other institutions either, e.g., in universities.[25] In the absence of the conditions that are necessary for authority, we ought to look for other ways of working together.

As an alternative, we might try to find more "democratic" procedures, procedures involving mutual counseling, consultation, and collaboration. Mutual accommodation and persuasion should take the place of one person issuing commands to others below. In the long run, such methods are the only ones that can hold up under rational scrutiny in situations in which there is a divergence of goals, concerns, and interests, but where there is still a modicum of goodwill.

NOTES

1. This essay was originally presented in response to Professor Saul Touster's "Decision-Making in the Nurse/Physician Relationship: Authority, Obedience and Collaboration," a paper presented at a conference on "Nursing and the Humanities: A Public Dialogue," held at the University of Connecticut Health Center, Farmington, November, 1977.

2. According to the dictionary, quandary refers "to the subjective aspect of a dilemma and emphasizes perplexity and vacillation."

3. By a "moral dilemma" I mean an unavoidable situation in which one is forced to choose between performing one obligation rather than another, or to choose between evils, rights or wrongs, duties, and so on. A good example of a moral dilemma in this sense is having to choose between saving a person's life and telling a lie. In philosophical jargon, a dilemma represents a clash between prima facie duties. As I have argued elsewhere, there are many other kinds of ethical problems besides those arising from dilemmas. See my "The Task of Ethics," in Warren Reich (ed.), *The Encyclopedia of Bioethics*, New York: Macmillan, 1978, vol. 1, pp. 400-07.

4. See Burton J. Bledstein, *The Culture of Professionalism: The Middle Class and the Development of Higher Education in America*. New York: Norton, 1977. Strictly speaking, nursing lacks some of the essential perquisites of a profession, as Touster points out.

5. See Bertrand de Jouvenal, *Sovereignty* (trans. J. F. Huntington). Chicago: University of Chicago Press, 1957, p. 32. In calling it a capacity, I want to stress the counterfactual aspect of power. Frequently, there is no need for a person with power to exercise that power, e.g., the power that goes with a gun, because the desires and preferences of the parties in fact coincide or they obey out of habit. Such is the case with charismatic power, for example. But power, in the sense of might, usually comes into play in marginal cases, since it is generally not the most effective way of controlling the behavior of others. Obviously, a great deal more needs to be said about power. It should be stressed that here we are concerned with power only in the narrow political and social sense and a sense that makes it possible to differentiate between the power of a doctor or administrator and his authority.

6. H.L.A. Hart, *The Concept of Law*. Oxford: Clarendon Press, 1961, p. 20.

7. de Jouvenal, *Sovereignty*, p. 33.

8. See Hobbes's distinction between counsel and command: "Now counsel is a precept in which the reason of my obeying it, is taken from the thing itself which is advised; but command is a precept, in which the cause of my obedience depends on the will of the commander." *De Cive*, S. P. Lamprecht (ed.), New York: Appleton-Century Crofts, 1949, p. 155.

9. See Richard B. Friedman, "On the concept of authority in political philosophy," reprinted in Richard E. Flathman, (ed.), *Concepts in Social and Political Philosophy*, New York: Macmillan, 1973, especially pp. 127 ff.

10. It makes no difference whether the claimant claims the authority for someone else or for himself.

11. The point is a logical or ethical one; in the absence of reasons for accepting a person as an authority, his alleged authority reduces to power, brute power, if you will.

12. See note 3, *supra*. Elsewhere, I call this kind of dilemma a "conflict of obligations." See my "Remarks on the conflict of obligations," *Journal of Philosophy*, September 11, 1958.

13. Inasmuch as totally dependent human beings, e.g., infants and idiots, cannot have obligations, the concept of authority has no immediate applicability to them.

14. Perhaps this consideration points to one way of distinguishing between power and authority; power can be unlimited, authority cannot. The power of a kidnapper over a captive often is close to being unlimited.

15. The *locus classicus* for an argument aimed at establishing the limits of authority is John Locke's *A Letter Concerning Toleration*. New York: Liberal Arts Press, Bobbs-Merrill, 1950. Locke argues that legislation regarding religion is impermissible because it is not authorized in the original contract establishing the civil authority.

16. Logically the two possible types of moral argumentation involve the difference between what may be called "refutation" and "confutation." Showing that you have no duty to do x, i.e., refuting the claim, must be distinguished logically from showing that you have a duty not to do x, i.e., confuting the claim. See my "The issue of relativism," in John Ladd, (ed.), *Ethical Relativism*. Belmont, California: Wadsworth, 1973.

17. I assume that "to obey" is to comply with a *command* in contradistinction to complying with a request, a piece of advice or other kinds of guidance. See Hobbes's distinction quoted above in note 8.

18. For a critique of the concept of ethics as a *technē*, see my "Egalitarianism and elitism in ethics," *L'Egalité*, V, Brussels, 1978.

19. Simply *saying* so is not sufficient to make it true.

20. For a critique of this notion, see my "Legal and moral obligation," in J. Roland Pennock and John Chapman, (eds.), *NOMOS XII: Political and Moral Obligation*. New York: Atherton Press, 1970.

21. There is, as far as I know, no standard use for these terms in discussions of authority by philosophers and political theorists.

22. We shall see that this difference may be crucial in the present inquiry, for nurses and doctors often have different goals in mind with regard to a patient,

and the patient himself may have a different goal from that of the doctor or that of the nurse.

23. For more on this concept of morality, see my *The Structure of a Moral Code*, Cambridge, Mass.: Harvard University Press, 1957.

24. Elsewhere I have expressed some reservations about these kinds of obligation, but they are immaterial to the present issue. See my "Legal and moral obligation," in J. Roland Pennock and John Chapman, (eds.), *NOMOS XII: Political and Moral Obligation*. New York: Atherton Press, 1970.

25. The decline of authority in our society has been called the "eclipse" or the "twilight" of authority.

9

Three Models of the
Nurse-Patient Relationship

Sheri Smith

A critical philosophical issue about nursing is raised in several of the essays in this volume, but it has been left unresolved. That issue is the question of the nature of the nurse-patient relationship. The failure to resolve the issue is critical, for the solution of ethical dilemmas in nursing practice often depends upon the definition of nursing and the responsibilities and rights thought to be inherent in the nurse-patient relationship.[1] My purpose in this chapter is to characterize three views of the nature of the nurse-patient relationship—the surrogate mother, nurse technician, and contracted clinician models—and to show the strengths and weaknesses of those models and their consequences for nursing practice. I will contend that assumptions about the nature of the nurse-patient relationship pervade the discussion of ethical dilemmas in nursing practice. In order to support that contention I will use examples from the essays by Dan Brock, who argues for the contracted clinician model; Mila Aroskar, who discusses the surrogate mother model in commenting on historical images of nurses; and Sally Gadow, whose conceptualizations of nursing can be shown to provide a philosophical basis for the models presented herein. My discussion of nursing models owes much to Robert Veatch's description of analogous models for the patient-physician relationship.[2] The question of how far the analogy between nurse-patient and physician-patient relationships can be drawn, and how the nature of the nurse-patient relationship might be altered by the relationship the patient has with his physician, is one on which I will comment briefly at the end of this discussion.

THE NURSE AS SURROGATE MOTHER

We can distinguish the three major models of the nurse-patient relationship by their conceptualizations of the extent and nature of the nurse's ethical responsibility and the assumptions made concerning patients and illness. In the surrogate mother model the nurse's primary responsibility and commitment is to the patient. (It should be noted here that, for the purposes of this discussion, "patient" will be understood to mean a competent adult.) The ethical responsibility of the nurse is defined by this commitment to the patient, as it is spelled out in nursing codes of ethics such as the American Nurses' Association Code. The nurse is even urged by the ANA code to serve as protector of the patient when his care and safety are in jeopardy through the actions of others. Other ethical responsibilities which nurses have, for example, in relation to physicians, are derived from this primary commitment to the patient.

It is the model of the nurse as a surrogate mother which has exerted greatest influence in the history of nursing and nursing education.[3] On this model, the nurse's ethical responsibility is understood as an unlimited commitment to the patient. It is the nurse's obligation to provide nursing care, to take care of the patient, and to act in his or her best interests at all times. The nurse has ultimate responsibility for the care which the patient receives. This means that the nurse also has an obligation to determine what constitutes the best care for the patient, and to act in his or her behalf if that care is not being provided. The nurse, then, has a kind of total commitment to patient care and ultimate responsiblity for determining that the patient's best interests are served.

However, this commitment to the patient alone would not give rise to the surrogate mother model. It is only when joined with observa-

tions about the nature of sickness and patients that the model is derived. Patients, generally, are sick, suffering, fearful, dependent individuals. Because of illness and hospitalization, patients may be unable to exercise emotional control or to make important decisions,
and, in at least some respects, may be irrational.[4] Consequently, the
patient cannot be trusted to make the best decisions about his or her
care, if able to make decisions at all. The patient needs someone to
provide care and to make the decisions, i.e., decisions for his or her
own good. The nurse's commitment to care for the patient, then, is a
commitment to an individual who is sick, dependent, and perhaps
unable to understand what his or her best interests are. The nurse's
relationship to the patient should be that of a surrogate mother to her
child.

It should be noted here that, on this model, the values of the nurse
carry great weight, since nurses will make critical decisions in terms of
their own values, i.e., their ideas about what constitutes the best interests of the patient. For example, a nurse might attempt to persuade
a patient to accept a treatment for the patient's own good. She might
withhold information if she believed that a patient would make the
"wrong" choice if the information were provided. She might even
make decisions concerning the appropriate goals for a patient's treatment. In short, acting on her responsibility for the care of the patient,
the nurse may impose her own judgments and decisions about care.

On this model, then, the nurse's concern for the patient's welfare
and intervention in his life are similar to a parent's concern for a child's
welfare and intervention in the child's life. It is this conceptualization
of nursing that is revealed by the stereotype of the nurse as mother
described by Mila Aroskar in her essay "The Fractured Image: The
Public Stereotype of Nursing and the Nurse." She suggests that traditionally nursing has implied a mother's relationship to her children,
caring for her family and managing her home.[5] Moreover, Aroskar
points out, in the first American nursing schools, the family was the
model for the hospital, a model in which the nurse is seen as mother,
the physician as father, and patients as children.[6]

In her comments on the image of the nurse Aroskar supports the
conclusions of JoAnn Ashley in *Hospitals, Paternalism, and the Role
of the Nurse.* Ashley observes, "The role of women (nurses) was very

early conceived as that of caring for the 'hospital family.' Their purpose was to provide efficient economical production in the form of patient care; they were to be loyal to the institution and devoted to preserving its reputation. Through service and self-sacrifice, they were to work continuously to keep the 'family' happy . . . Like mothers in a household, nurses were responsible for meeting the needs of all members of the hospital 'family'—from patients to physicians."[7]

Thus, traditionally, the "mother" image has been the prevailing image of the nurse. The corresponding philosophical assumption is that the nature of the nurse-patient relationship is fundamentally like that of a mother to a child. This assumption has had profound impact on our beliefs about the character of nursing dilemmas, and our expectations concerning appropriate solutions of ethical issues in nursing practice, for it includes the belief that the nurse should always act in what is perceived to be the patient's interest.

This belief, that the nurse should always act in the patient's interest, as Sally Gadow points out, implies a conceptualization of nursing as paternalism. She notes that paternalism is often defended as the belief that, for an individual's own good, decisions should be made by those most capable of knowing what is in his best interest.[8] In actuality, however, paternalistic acts and attitudes limit the rights or freedom of individuals in their own interests.[9] Paternalism this involves the intent to obtain what is believed to be a good for the other person, with the effect of violating his known wishes.[10] To accept the surrogate mother model of the nurse-patient relationship, therefore, with its assumptions about the extent of the nurse's ethical responsibility to the patient, and the helplessness and need of the patient, is to conceive of nursing as paternalism.

THE NURSE AS TECHNICIAN

If the two primary assumptions of the surrogate mother model concerning the extent of the nurse's ethical responsibility and the nature of patients are rejected, the resulting model of the nurse-patient relationship is a view which could be called the technical model. This model is derived from the contemporary view of nursing as a clinical science.[11]

The nurse, it is suggested, should provide scientific care; that is, the nurse should apply scientific methods and scientific treatment to the care of patients. The nurse's commitment to the patient is a commitment to provide the best nursing care possible, meeting the patient's needs to the best of her ability. Further, the nurse is committed to the objective, nonjudgmental, noninterfering application of nursing knowledge and skills in treating patients. The nurse must respect the values and beliefs of patients, and be fair and unbiased in the treatment of patients. A nurse should not impose her own values or make value judgments in administering nursing care; on the contrary, she must remain ethically neutral. Thus the extent of the nurse's ethical responsibility is limited to the correct application of knowledge and skills to meet the needs of the patient.

The needs of the patient are biological phenomena with which a nurse must deal factually and objectively by providing care as requested by the patient. It is assumed that the patient's ability to make decisions and to judge his own best interests is not impaired by illness or hospitalization. Consequently, the patient retains ultimate responsibility for identifying his needs and determining his best interests. The nurse has no role in determining those interests and needs, either by attempting to influence the patient, or by refusing to help him attain his goals.

If the patient is regarded as completely capable of making his own decisions about what is good for him, and the nurse's obligation to the patient is to provide the scientific care he requests (or the physician requests for him), then the model of the nurse-patient relationship is as follows. It is a relationship between a technician, the nurse, and an individual who receives technical assistance, the patient. The nurse should merely apply knowledge and technical skills as requested by the patient. Her only concern as a professional should be to apply those skills correctly and objectively. That is to say, she should not be concerned with the decisions which the patient might make about his treatment or health, even if her involvement in his decisions would be for the patient's own good.[12] She should just provide the patient with any information and technical advice which he needs in order to make decisions concerning his health. It is a consequence of this model that the nurse would simply supply nursing care as requested, regardless of the foolishness or moral repugnance of the patient's requests and decisions. The nurse's moral values and judgments would be irrelevant to her function as a provider of nursing care.[13]

Belief in the nurse's ethical neutrality, her concern and obligation to provide the best, correct care, and the unimpaired rational abilities of the patient produce this model of the nurse-patient relationship. If the nurse's responsibility on this model is construed to include protecting the patient's interests as he has determined them, then the nurse's role is to serve as an advocate for the patient. This image of nursing as technical assistance to patients is the conceptualization which Gadow calls consumerism.[14]

THE NURSE AS CONTRACTED CLINICIAN

The third model of the nurse-patient relationship follows from the assumption that the patient is capable of determining his own best interests, a premise about patients which is also assumed by the technical model, and the belief that the ethical responsibility of the nurse is defined by the rights of the patient. The patient's right to self-determination is essential to the rights-based moral view of the nurse-patient relationship which Dan Brock develops in his essay "The Nurse-Patient Relation: Some Rights and Duties." Brock argues that a nurse's unique relation to the patient can be explained only by viewing the nurse-patient relationship as arising from an agreement between nurse and patient, an agreement in which the patient contracts to have specified care provided by the nurse and the nurse incurs an obligation to the patient to provide that care.[15] On this model of the nurse-patient relationship, the patient has the right to control both what happens to his body and the role which the nurse takes with him in providing nursing care;[16] ". . . the right to determine what is done to and for the patient, and to control, within broad limits, the course of the patient's treatment and care, originates and generally remains with the patient."[17] Thus the nurse's commitment to the patient is a commitment to provide the nursing care which he chooses. Nurses are not justified in doing something because it is in the best interests of the patient, moreover, since the right to act in the patient's interest is ". . . *created* and *limited* by the permission or consent (from the patient-nurse/

physician agreement) the patient has given."[18] Therefore, it is the patient's right to control the course of his treatment, his right to self-determination, which defines the ethical responsibility of the nurse.

An important consequence of the contracted clinician model is that the nurse is not required to be ethically neutral. Since the nurse-patient relationship arises from an agreement, the nurse can refuse to participate in the relationship, if her own ethical values would be compromised. For example, the nurse can refuse to care for abortion patients if she believes abortion is unethical. Therefore, the nurse's commitment to the patient is limited by her own permission or consent as well as by the rights of the patient.

The patient's right to self-determination, which is essential in this model, is also essential for Sally Gadow's conceptualization of nursing as existential advocacy. This conceptualization is based on the belief that "freedom of self-determination is the most fundamental and valuable human right, and therefore is a greater good than any which health care can provide."[19] Nurses must assist patients in authentically exercising that freedom of self-determination, that is, in making decisions which express the full complexity of their values.[20] The nurse is obligated to act in the patient's interest, but she cannot define what the patient's "best interest" is. She must assist patients to determine their best interests and to become clear about what they want to do.[21] "Existential advocacy, as the essence of nursing, is the nurse's participation with the patient in determining the unique meaning which the experience of health, illness, suffering, or dying is to have for that individual."[22]

Gadow argues for existential advocacy as the philosophical foundation of nursing. This conceptualization of nursing supports Brock's model of the nurse-patient relationship in its central features. Both Brock and Gadow agree that the fundamental value to be preserved in the nurse-patient relationship is the patient's right to self-determination. They are agreed that the patient determines what his best interests are and that the patient has the right to decide which role the nurse takes with him.[23] The conceptualization of nursing as advocacy, in Gadow's sense, could therefore serve as a basis for the contracted clinician model of the nurse-patient relationship. It is important to note here that it is not patients' rights advocacy which supports the contracted clinician model. For, as Gadow suggests, patients' rights advocacy is really what she calls consumerism, that is, the belief that the nurse should just obey the patient's wishes. Consumerism thus forces the patient to make a decision autonomously. It involves the paternalistic assumption that patients should make important decisions with only technical assistance and information.[24] However, Brock and Gadow both argue that the patient's right to self-determination is inviolate. That is, it is the patient's right to determine what he needs from the nurse; whether he makes a decision autonomously is his choice. The patient can, if he wishes, receive advice from the nurse; he can even choose a paternalistic relationship with the nurse. The patient's freedom to determine his relationship with the nurse is the key to the contracted clinician model.

AN ETHICAL DILEMMA

I have attempted to show that different beliefs about the ethical responsibilities of nurses and assumptions about patients yield three models of the nurse-patient relationship. These models have implications for nursing practice which are of critical importance. I will argue that, on the basis of these ethical implications, the contracted clinician model should be accepted. In order to establish that, it will be necessary to consider an example. The implications for nursing practice will be most clearly revealed if we consider a case which will show the essential differences concerning the responsibility of the nurse with regard to the patient's best interests, and the role of the nurse's personal values and beliefs.

Mr. A. is a 56-year-old man who has had leukemia for one year. He has again voluntarily admitted himself for control of hemorrhaging and intractable pain. He also suffers from very high fevers and an oral infection with open sores. He is depressed and anxious about the future. During the past six months he has been hospitalized frequently to receive chemotherapy and blood transfusions. On recent hospitalizations, however, the chemotherapy has been discontinued because of Mr. A.'s lowered white blood count. Though he is aware of his deteriorating condition, he is optimistic about the possibility of another remission.

When he is examined by the physician, the physician informs him that he is in the terminal phase of leukemia. The physician explains that he will receive painkillers and will be treated with intravenous fluids to combat the dehydration. Blood transfusions and a bone marrow aspiration will also be used to stabilize the progress of the disease. The physician, however, does not hold out any hope of prolonging Mr. A.'s life for a significant period of time. He indicates that there is only a remote hope of remission.

Mr. A., extremely upset at this prognosis, exclaims that he cannot bear the pain any longer, and expresses a wish to die. Mr. A. explains his situation to his family, and again expresses his wish to die without any prolonged suffering. Mrs. A. disagrees vehemently with him, and argues that any means available should be used to prolong Mr. A.'s life.

Consequently, Mr. A. is admitted to the hospital, the intravenous treatment is begun, and he is left to rest. Several minutes later Nurse B., who has been present throughout Mr. A.'s examination and treatment, enters his room to discover that Mr. A. is unconscious; the flow of intravenous fluids has been mistakenly adjusted so that all of the intravenous fluids have been absorbed. As a result it is very unlikely that Mr. A. will regain consciousness. Moreover, the rapid infusion of the fluids will have immediate fatal consequences if action is not taken. What should Nurse B. do?[25]

As with all case descriptions, there is some ambiguity in this situation. It is unclear why Mr. A. voluntarily admitted himself under the circumstances or why he consented to the treatment. Since there are many aspects of this case that deserve more careful description and analysis, it cannot be adequately discussed within the scope of this chapter. It will serve, however, to illustrate the ethical implications of the three nurse-patient models.

It is necessary for the purposes of clarifying the implications of these models to make an assumption about the judgments and personal moral values of Nurse B. Let us assume that she disagrees with Mr. A.; she is convinced Mr. A. has valuable life remaining, and she believes that preserving life is a duty. In this situation there are essentially two options open to Nurse B. Nurse B. can respect Mr. A.'s wish to die and refrain from initiating any treatment, or Nurse B. can do everything possible to keep Mr. A. alive—for example, she can page the physician and immediately begin extraordinary emergency procedures. The critical element in Nurse B.'s decision in this case will be her own philosophical view of the nature of the nurse-patient relationship, that is, the role which she believes her values should play in that relationship, as well as her beliefs about her ethical responsibility for the patient.

If Nurse B. assumes the surrogate mother model of the nurse-patient relationship, there are important consequences for her practice of nursing. The strength of this model is that it clearly recognizes the vulnerability, suffering, and need of the patient. It recognizes that patients may not make the best decisions in situations such as Mr. A.'s situation. Nurse B., consequently, will be aware of Mr. A.'s vulnerability; she will be sympathetic, understanding, and willing to provide the mothering care and concern which Mr. A. may need.

Moreover, Nurse B. will regard her ethical commitment to the patient, Mr. A., as an all-encompassing responsibility to do what she believes is in Mr. A.'s best interests. Consequently, in this situation, she will act according to her perception of what is best for Mr. A. Even though Mr. A. has expressed a wish to die, she will page the physician and initiate emergency procedures in an attempt to save Mr. A.'s life.

If Nurse B. accepts the technical model, on the other hand, her action in this situation will be quite different. On the technical model, Nurse B.'s own beliefs about the sanctity of life are irrelevant, since she is required to be ethically neutral in her practice of nursing. Her skills are to be utilized to satisfy the patient's wishes and requests. If a patient requests an abortion, for example, the nurse's obligation is to supply good nursing care, regardless of her own judgments about the desirability or morality of abortion. In this case, since Mr. A. has expressed a wish to die, Nurse B. would ignore her own judgment about the best interests of Mr. A. and the immorality of letting him die. Nurse B. has no obligation to undertake any actions aimed at saving his life, for Mr. A. clearly does not wish to have his life saved. Therefore, Nurse B. will not initiate treatment.

Similarly, if Nurse B. accepts the contracted clinician model, she will not initiate treatment. On this model her ethical responsibility will be defined by Mr. A.'s right to control and determine what happens to him. Though Nurse B. disagrees with Mr. A.'s wish to die, she will not impose her own judgments and values in this situation. She will allow Mr. A. to die.

The differences between the technical model and the contracted clinician model are not obvious in this case, for though they involve quite different assumptions, they result in the same action. The key difference between these models is the role of the nurse's values in the nurse-patient relationship. On the technical model, the nurse's values are irrelevant, for she must remain ethically neutral. However, on the contracted clinician model, the nurse's values are important factors in the relationship with the patient. The nurse can refuse to participate in that relationship if her values are compromised. Thus this model allows the nurse's values to become an important aspect of the relationship with the patient.

Only the general features of the surrogate mother, technical, and contracted clinician models of the nurse-patient relationship have been outlined here. However, some significant conclusions can be drawn. First, the surrogate-mother model of the nurse-patient relationship is inadequate for the same reasons that a paternalistic model of the physician-patient relationship is unacceptable, i.e., it condones actions which violate a patient's right to self-determination. It is clearly ethically objectionable for the nurse to impose her beliefs about the patient's best interests and in effect to make an important decision for the patient. Secondly, it seems evident to me that the technical model is also inadequate. The nurse, in caring for patients and making decisions about nursing care, is not functioning solely as a technician. An acceptable model for the nurse-patient relationship must recognize the ethical aspects of nursing practice.

Because it recognizes the ethical aspects of nursing practice and the patient's right to self-determination, the contracted clinician model is the best of these three models. There is, however, one consequence of this which deserves comment. As Brock points out, the implication of his model is that the nurse-patient relationship is essentially the same as the physician-patient relationship. It seems to me, though, that there is a significant difference. Though both nurse and physician are viewed as having a contractual relationship with the patient, there is an additional factor which complicates the nurse-patient relationship. The nurse is obligated to provide nursing care because of her agreement with the patient; furthermore, she is also obligated to obey the physician because of her agreement with the patient. That is, this obligation is imposed by the agreement with the patient because the nurse agrees to provide the nursing care necessary to the patient's needs as he or she identifies them. She is therefore obligated to assist the physician in providing care necessary to the patient's needs. The physician, however, does not have a similar obligation to the nurse. This suggests to me that these relationships may be significantly different in some respects. The question of how the nature of the nurse-patient relationship is altered by the relationship the patient has with his physician is an issue which deserves careful analysis, for these relationships are central to some of the most difficult ethical dilemmas in nursing practice.

NOTES

1. Sally Gadow argues that nursing can be defined in terms of the nurse-patient relationship. See chapter 4 of this volume, "Existential Advocacy: Philosophical Foundation of Nursing."

2. Robert Veatch discusses his models of the patient-physician relationship in "Models for Ethical Medicine in a Revolutionary Age," *Hastings Center Report*, June 1972, pp. 5-7.

3. The influence of this image of nurses as surrogate mothers has been reported by several nurses and sociologists. For example, Hans O. Mauksch, "Nursing: Churning for Change," in Freeman, Howard E., *et. al* (eds.), *Handbook of Medical Sociology*, 2nd ed., Englewood Cliffs, N.J.: Prentice-Hall, Inc., 1972, and most recently Myra E. Levine in "Nursing Ethics and the Ethical Nurse," *American Journal of Nursing*, May 1977, p. 845.

4. Some interesting observations concerning patients are made by Henry J. Lederer, "How the Sick View Their World," in *The Journal of Social Issues*, 8(4), 1952, pp. 4-15.

5. Mila Aroskar, in chapter 2 of this volume, "The Fractured Image: The Public Stereotype of Nursing and the Nurse."

6. *Ibid.*

7. JoAnn Ashley, *Hospitals, Paternalism, and the Role of the Nurse*, New York: Teachers College Press, 1976, p. 17.

8. Gadow, "Existential Advocacy."

9. *Ibid.*

10. *Ibid.*

11. The view presented here about the nature of the nurse-patient relationship is that expressed by Gerene Major in her paper "The Abortion Patient and the Nurse." My thinking concerning the issues discussed herein was developed in response to her paper.

12. Gadow, "Existential Advocacy."

13. *Ibid.*

14. *Ibid.*

15. Dan Brock, in chapter 5 of this volume, "The Nurse-Patient Relation: Some Rights and Duties."

16. *Ibid.*

17. *Ibid.*

18. *Ibid.*

19. Gadow, "Existential Advocacy."

20. *Ibid.*

21. *Ibid.*

22. *Ibid.*

23. Gadow believes that the patient and nurse can freely decide what their relationship will be.

24. *Ibid.*

25. This case is based upon a case presented to me by Gertrude Mulvey, R.N.

Index